MW01488812

Telephone Numbers

Emergency Medical Service (EMS): _____ Campus Security: _____

Fire: _____ Police: _____ Local Poison Control: _____

National Suicide Prevention Lifeline: _800.273.8255_ National Poison Control: _800.222.1222_

Community Urgent Care Center: _____ Campus Urgent Care: _____

Student Health Services: _____ After Hours Number: _____

Student Counseling/Mental Health Services: _____

Personal Physician: _____

Nearest Hospital: _____ Pharmacy: _____

Health Insurance Information

Company: _____ Phone Number: _____

Address: _____

Policyholder's Name: _____ Policy Number: _____

What to Tell Your Health Care Provider

(Use this summary when you call or visit a health care provider.)

Symptoms

- ❏ Pain (location and severity)
- ❏ Fever/chills
- ❏ Skin problems (location and description)
- ❏ Eye, ear, nose, throat problems

- ❏ Stomach problems
- ❏ Nausea/vomiting
- ❏ Breathing problems
- ❏ Anxiety, depression

- ❏ Duration of symptoms
- ❏ Constant or intermittent
- ❏ Things that make symptoms better or worse

Other problems: _____

Specific questions I have now: _____

What I need to do: _____

Medications

	Name/Dose	Name/Dose
Prescribed and over-the-counter medications I take:	_____	_____
Herbs and supplements I take:	_____	_____
Medications I'm allergic to:	_____	_____

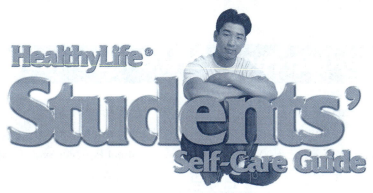

HealthyLife® Students' Self-Care Guide

by Don R. Powell, Ph.D.

and the American Institute for Preventive Medicine

Note: This book is not meant to substitute for expert medical advice or treatment. The information is given to help you make informed choices about your health. Follow your doctor's or health care provider's advice if it differs from what is given in this book.

Understand that many of the designations used by manufacturers and sellers to distinguish their products are claimed as trademarks. Where those designations appear in this book and the American Institute for Preventive Medicine was aware of a trademark claim, the designations have been printed in capital letters (e.g., Tylenol).

This guide is one of a series of publications, programs, and online products, developed by the American Institute for Preventive Medicine, designed to help individuals reduce health care costs and improve the quality of their lives. We publish a companion student mental health self-care guide called Minding Your Mental Health. We also provide many wellness and disease management publications and programs.

For more information, call or write:	**For free health information:**
American Institute for Preventive Medicine 30445 Northwestern Hwy., Suite 350 Farmington Hills, MI 48334 248.539.1800 / Fax 248.539.1808 email: aipm@healthylife.com	Access: www.HealthyLearn.com. At this site, type a topic in the box for "Search MedlinePlus."

{*Note:* "LifeArt image copyright, Williams & Wilkins. All rights reserved" applies to illustrations in this book noted with a single *.}

ISBN-10   0-9635612-0-0   ISBN-13   978-09635612-0-0

Contributors and Reviewers

A. Nancy Anderson, R.N.C., B.S.N., Nurse Director, College of Wooster Student Health Center, Wooster, OH

Julie Bloomquist, B.A., Baker College, Owosso, MI

Ronda Bokram, M.S., R.D., Nutritionist, Health Education Services, Olin Health Center, Michigan State University, East Lansing, MI

Rosetta M. Brown-Greaney, R.N.C., M.S.N., Director/Nurse Practitioner, Crandall Health Center at Alfred University, Alfred, NY

James Cowan, P.A.-L., Physician Assistant, Olin Health Center, Michigan State University, East Lansing, MI

Dee W. Edington, Ph.D., Director, Health Management Research Center, University of Michigan, Division of Kinesiology, Ann Arbor, MI

Bill Hettler, M.D., Director, Health Services, University of Wisconsin-Stevens Point, Stevens Point, WI

Stephen J. Hughs, M.D., Associate Director for Clinical Services, Gannett University Health Center, Cornell University, Ithaca, NY

Illinois State University Body Acceptance Coalition, (submitted by Nikki Gegel, M.S., Chairperson), Normal, IL

Khaleelah Aisha Jones, Research Assistant & Full Time Student, Michigan State University, East Lansing, MI

Jeanette Karwan, R.D., Director, Product Development, American Institute for Preventive Medicine

Jonathon B. Kermict, M.A., C.H.E.S., Health Educator, Fitness & Exercise, Michigan State University, East Lansing, MI

Travis Lairson, Patient Advocate, Student Wellness Center, Ohio State University, Columbus, OH

Dennis P. Martell, Ph.D., Health Educator, Olin Health Center, Michigan State University, East Lansing, MI

Amanda McPhail, Student, Western Michigan University, Kalamazoo, MI

John D. McPhail, C.R.C., L.P.C., President, Wisdom to Wellness, Inc., Okemos, MI

Jordan S. Powell, J.D., Associate, Levin & Perconti, Chicago, IL, B.A. University of Michigan, Ann Arbor, MI

S.J. Rajan, Staff Physician, Olin Health Center, Michigan State University, East Lansing, MI

Tom Ryan, M.D., Medical Director, Virginia Tech Schiffert Health Center, Blacksburg, VA

Mary Kaye Sawyer-Morse, Ph.D., R.D., Associate Professor of Nutrition, University of the Incarnate Word, San Antonio, TX

Naomi A. Shaheen, M.Ed., Former Vice-President, Business Development, American Institute for Preventive Medicine

Michael W. Straus, P.A., Physician Assistant & Certified Athletic Trainer, Michigan State University, East Lansing, MI

David F. Szewczyk, R.N., Medical Writer, St. Clair Shores, MI

Rosie C. Taylor, M.S., R.N., A.N.P., Director of Health Services, Sweet Briar College, Sweet Briar, VA

Mary Trieste, B.S.N., R.N., Director, Health Education, Empire BlueCross BlueShield, New York, NY

Andria Watha, Graphic Designer, American Institute For Preventive Medicine

Mia Flor Wimberly, Medical Student, Michigan State University, East Lansing, MI

Table of Contents

Introduction

You are at a time in your life when you need to make a lot of decisions: Decisions on career choices, future plans and goals, etc. You need to make decisions to take care of your health, too. Knowing what to do can be confusing. You may not have had many health problems in the past, and when you did, your parents probably took care of you. You need to fend for yourself now. This guide can help. It contains 3 sections. The first one addresses 21 common health problems. The second section covers issues that deal with keeping you safe while keeping you healthy. The third section presents information on lifestyle issues. Like a roommate or a friend, this self-care guide can come to your aid when you need it. It may even save your life!

Section I – Common Health Problems

How to Use This Section

■ Find the health problem in Section I of the Table of Contents and go to that page. The problems are listed in order from A to Z.

■ Read about the problem, its symptoms, what causes it (if known), and treatments.

■ Scrutinize the "Questions to Ask." Start at the top of the flowchart and answer YES or NO to each question.

How to Use This Section, *Continued*

Follow the arrows in the flowchart until you get to one of these answers:

Get Immediate Care

You should get help immediately. If symptoms threaten life, go to a hospital emergency department, if you can do so quickly and safely. If not, call 9-1-1 or your local rescue squad. Symptoms that threaten life include:

- No breathing.
- Unconsciousness.
- Difficulty breathing.
- Severe bleeding.
- Head or neck injury.
- Suicidal or homicidal intent.
- Choking.

For symptoms that don't threaten life, immediate care means seeing your health care provider or going to an urgent care center right away. If your school has a health service center, find out where it is and when it is open. Find out where to go for urgent care, both on and off campus. Make sure you know phone numbers for these places and write them on page 1.

Find out, now, how your health insurance covers medical emergencies when you are in the state you live in, when you are out of state, and even out of the country. Then you'll know what to do if a health problem occurs. You may need to get additional insurance when you travel or study abroad.

See Provider

Call your health care provider. State the problem(s) so it can be determined how soon you need to be seen. The term "provider" can be used for a number of health care providers. They include:

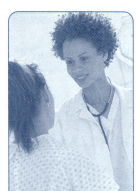

Be open and honest when you talk to a health care provider.

- Your primary doctor, physician's assistant (P.A.), nurse practitioner (N.P.), etc.
- Doctors, registered nurses, and counselors at your school's Health Service or Mental Health Service.
- Walk-in clinic health care providers.

Call Provider

Call your health care provider and state the problem. You will be given advice on what to do.

Use Self-Care

You can probably take care of the problem yourself if you answered NO to all questions in the flowcharts. Use the self-care items that are listed, but call your health care provider if you don't feel better soon. You may have some other problem.

To learn more about topics covered in this guide and other health issues, access the Web site listed on the back cover of this book and www.cdc.gov/features/collegehealth.

Abdominal Pain

"When I got to school, my stomach did a lot of backflips because of all of the new foods. I miss my mom's cooking."

John L., Notre Dame University

The abdomen is the body region between the lower ribs and the pelvis that contains many vital organs:

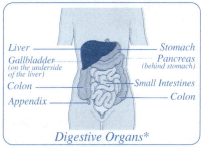

Liver — Gallbladder *(on the underside of the liver)* — Colon — Appendix — Stomach — Pancreas *(behind stomach)* — Small Intestines — Colon

Digestive Organs*

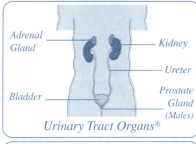

Adrenal Gland — Bladder — Kidney — Ureter — Prostate Gland *(Males)*

Urinary Tract Organs*

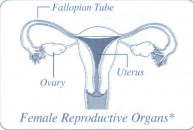

Fallopian Tube — Uterus — Ovary

Female Reproductive Organs*

Abdominal pain can range from mild to severe: be dull or sharp; acute or chronic. Acute pain is sudden pain. Chronic pain can be constant or pain that recurs over time. The type of pain, its location, and other symptoms that come with it, help suggest the cause.

Signs, Symptoms & Causes

There are many causes of abdominal pain. Common ones in students and the symptoms that accompany them are listed below.

Constipation

Constipation results from not drinking enough fluids, not eating enough dietary fiber, not being active enough, and from misusing laxatives. Symptoms of constipation are:

- A hard time passing stool, not being able to pass stool, and/or having very hard stools.
- Straining to have a bowel movement.
- Abdominal swelling or feeling of continued fullness after passing stool.

Gastroenteritis

Gastroenteritis is inflammation of the lining of the stomach and intestines. Causes include having an intestinal virus, food poisoning, and drinking contaminated water or too much alcohol. Symptoms of gastroenteritis include:

- Abdominal pain or cramping.
- Nausea and/or vomiting.
- Diarrhea.
- Fever and/or chills.

It may be hard to tell from symptoms if you have an intestinal virus or food poisoning. Suspect food poisoning if others who have eaten the same foods you did also have symptoms.

Lactose Intolerance

Lactose intolerance results from a lack of an enzyme (lactase) needed to digest the sugar (lactose) in dairy products.

Abdominal Pain, *Continued*

Symptoms of lactose intolerance are:

- Abdominal cramping, pain, and bloating after drinking milk or eating other dairy products.
- Gas and diarrhea.

Menstrual Cramps in Females

Hormones cause the uterus to go into spasms. Premenstrual bloating increases the abdominal pain. Symptoms of menstrual cramps are:

- Mild to severe abdominal pain.
- Back pain, fatigue, and/or diarrhea.

Peptic Ulcer

A peptic ulcer is an ulcer in the stomach or first section of the small intestine. Symptoms include:

- A gnawing or burning pain between the breastbone and navel. This is the most common symptom. The pain often occurs between meals and in the morning. It may last from a few minutes to a few hours and may be relieved with taking an antacid.
- Loss of appetite and weight loss.
- Nausea or vomiting dark, red blood or material that looks like coffee grounds.
- Bloody, black, or tarry stools.

The 2 most common factors associated with peptic ulcers are:

- An infection with *Helicobacter pylori* (*H. pylori*) bacteria.
- The repeated use of aspirin and other nonsteroidal anti-inflammatory drugs (NSAIDs), such as over-the-counter and prescribed ibuprofen.

Peptic ulcers are not caused by stress, but stress can aggravate them. (See **"Stress"** on page 53.)

Treatment

Treatment depends on the cause. The key is knowing when it's just a minor problem like a mild stomach ache or when it's something worse. Pain that persists can be a sign of a medical condition or illness. Very severe abdominal pain usually requires immediate medical care.

Questions to Ask

Is the abdominal pain very severe or sudden, extreme, and constant? Is the pain so bad that you can't move or does it get a lot worse when you move?

YES Get Immediate Care

NO

Are all of these **symptoms of appendicitis** present?
- You have not had your appendix removed.
- Pain and tenderness that usually start in the upper part of the stomach or around the belly button and move to the lower right part of the abdomen. The pain can be sharp, severe, and felt more when the lower right abdomen is touched.
- Nausea, vomiting, or no appetite.
- Mild fever.

YES Get Immediate Care

NO

Flowchart continued on next page

Abdominal Pain, *Continued*

Flowchart continued

For females, do you have the following **signs and symptoms of an ectopic pregnancy or pelvic inflammatory disease (PID)**?
- You are sexually active and have missed one or more periods or have vaginal bleeding you can't explain.
- Cramping or pain that can be severe in your lower abdomen.
- Sudden fainting or dizziness.

YES Get Immediate Care

NO

Do you have **signs and symptoms of an acute kidney infection** listed on page 59?

YES Get Immediate Care

NO

Do you have the following **signs and symptoms of kidney stones**?
- The pain started in your side or back before it moved to your abdomen or groin.
- The pain can be constant or come and go. The pain may be severe.
- Your urine is bloody, cloudy, or dark-colored.
- Nausea and vomiting.
- Chills and fever, if you also have an infection. (See **Fever** on pages 33 and 34.)

YES See Provider

NO

Flowchart continued in next column

With abdominal pain, do you have any of these problems?
- The whites of your eyes or your skin looks yellow.
- Severe diarrhea or constipation lasts more than a week.
- Skin on the abdomen is sensitive.
- You have a bulge and/or discomfort (when pressed) anywhere on the abdomen.

YES See Provider

NO

Do you have **signs and symptoms of a bladder infection** listed on page 59?

YES See Provider

NO

With abdominal pain, are any of these problems present?
- Continued belching, nausea, gas, or gurgling noises.
- Pain worsens when you bend over or lie down.
- You could be pregnant.
- Menstrual cramps are severe enough to keep you from going to classes nearly every month.

YES Call Provider

NO

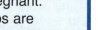 Use Self-Care

Self-Care

To Help Ease Pain in General

- Place a hot water bottle or a heating pad, set on low, over the area of pain.

- Find a comfortable position. Relax.

Abdominal Pain, *Continued*

■ Take an over-the-counter medicine for pain that does not cause stomach upset. (See "**Pain Relievers**" in "**Over-the-Counter Medication Safety**" on page 75.)

■ Don't wear tight-fitting clothes.

■ Don't do strenuous exercise.

■ Eat foods as tolerated.

For Constipation

■ Eat foods high in fiber: Bran; whole-grain breads and cereals; and fresh fruits and vegetables.

■ Drink at least 1¹/₂ to 2 quarts of water and other liquids every day. Hot water, tea, or coffee may help stimulate the bowel.

■ Get plenty of exercise.

■ Don't resist the urge to have a bowel movement.

■ If you take antacids or iron supplements and get constipated easily, discuss the use of these with your health care provider.

■ If needed, take an over-the-counter fiber supplement, such as Metamucil, or stool softener, such as Colace. Follow your health care provider's advice for the use of "stimulant" laxatives, such as Ex-Lax. Long-term use of them can make you even more constipated and lead to a mineral imbalance and reduced nutrient absorption.

For Food Poisoning

■ To prevent food poisoning:

  • Wash your hands and food preparation surfaces and utensils, especially after handling raw meat and eggs.

  • Cook foods to a safe temperature. Get information from: www.foodsafety.gov/keep/charts/mintemp.html

  • Refrigerate perishable foods promptly. These include milk, cheese, meat, poultry, eggs, and fish. Refrigerate leftovers, and use them within 3 to 4 days.

  • Hot foods should be kept at or above 140°F. Cold foods should be kept at or below 40°F. Carry items in a thermos or with a cold pack, if necessary.

  • When in doubt, throw it out.

■ When you have food poisoning, follow self-care measures in "**Vomiting & Nausea**" on page 66.

For Lactose Intolerance

See "**Self-Care for Lactose Intolerance**" on page 26.

For Menstrual Cramps

■ Take an over-the-counter medicine for pain. (See "**Pain Relievers**" in "**Over-the-Counter Medication Safety**" on page 75.)

■ Drink hot tea (regular, chamomile, or mint).

■ Hold a heating pad or hot water bottle on your abdomen or lower back.

■ Take a warm bath.

■ Gently massage your abdomen.

■ Do mild exercises, such as yoga and walking.

■ When you can, lie on your back and support your knees with a pillow.

■ Rest. Avoid stress as your period approaches.

{*Note:* If you get stomach aches due to stress, see "**Stress**" on pages 53 to 55 for information on how to deal with it.}

Acne

"Zits are the pits! I was hoping that by the time I got to college, my pimples would be gone. They weren't. I went to a dermatologist and did what he said. It's easier to look in the mirror now."

Sally J., Valparaiso University

Acne is a common skin condition. It occurs most often in teenagers and young adults, but can persist into adulthood.

Signs & Symptoms

The following occur on the face, neck, back, and/or shoulders:

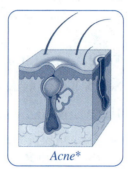

Acne*

- Whiteheads and/or blackheads.
- Red and painful pimples.
- Deeper lumps (cysts or nodules).

Causes & Risk Factors

Acne results when oil ducts below the skin get clogged. Factors that help cause acne include:

- Hormone changes during adolescence.
- Changes in hormone levels before a female's menstrual period or during pregnancy.
- Rich moisturizing lotions or oily makeup.
- Emotional stress.
- Nutritional supplements that have iodine.
- Some anticonvulsive medications (for seizures) and lithium (used to treat some forms of depression).

- Illegal (anabolic) steroids (used for muscle-building).

Foods and beverages, such as chocolate, nuts, greasy foods, and cola <u>do not cause</u> acne. If you find that eating certain foods make your acne worse, avoid them.

Treatment

Mild acne can be treated with self-care (see page 11). When this is not enough, a health care provider can prescribe one or more of the following:

- A topical cream medicine (retinoid) that contains an altered form of Vitamin A, such as Retin-A. {*Note:* Retin-A makes your skin more sensitive to the sun.}
- A topical cream, lotion, or wipe with an antibiotic, such as clindamycin or erythromycin.
- An antibiotic pill, such as doxycycline, minocycline, or tetracycline. {*Note:* These medicines can make birth control pills less effective and make your skin more sensitive to the sun.}
- For some females, a specific birth control pill.
- Isotretinoin. Brand names are Accutane Amnesteem, Claravis, and Sotret. This is usually prescribed for severe acne. {*Note:* Discuss this medicine with your health care provider. Females should not get pregnant while they take this medicine and for at least 1 month after stopping it, as it can cause severe birth defects. There is some evidence that pregnant females should avoid contact with sperm from males who take isotretinoin. Also, this medicine may cause depression, psychosis, and rarely, suicidal thoughts, suicide attempts, and suicide.}

Acne, *Continued*

Questions to Ask

Are you taking the medicine isotretinoin and are you planning suicide, making suicidal gestures, or do you have repeated thoughts of suicide or death?

YES → Get Immediate Care

NO

Is your acne very bad and do you have signs of an infection, such as a fever and swelling at the acne site?

YES → See Provider

NO

Do you have any of these problems?
• The acne results in scarring.
• The pimples are big and painful or widespread.
• The acne causes a lot of emotional embarrassment.

YES → Call Provider

NO

Have you tried self-care and it doesn't help or does it make your skin worse?

YES → Call Provider

NO

 Use Self-Care

Self-Care

- Gently wash your skin, where the acne appears, twice a day. Use a mild soap and clean washcloth. Work the soap into your skin gently for 1 to 2 minutes. Rinse well. **Don't scrub.**

- Wash after you exercise or sweat.

- Wash your hair at least every other day.

- For males: To soften your beard, wrap a warm towel around your face before you shave. Shave along the natural grain of the beard.

- Leave your skin alone! Don't squeeze, scratch, or poke at pimples. They can get infected and leave scars.

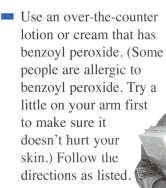

- Use an over-the-counter lotion or cream that has benzoyl peroxide. (Some people are allergic to benzoyl peroxide. Try a little on your arm first to make sure it doesn't hurt your skin.) Follow the directions as listed.

- Don't spend too much time in the sun, especially if you take antibiotics for acne. Don't use sun lamps.

- Use only oil-free and water-based makeup. Don't use greasy or oil-based creams, lotions, or makeup.

- If you take an antibiotic for acne treatment and get signs of a vaginal yeast infection (see page 61), use **"Self-Care For a Vaginal Yeast Infection"** on page 64.

For Information, Contact:

American Academy of Dermatology
888.462.DERM (462.3376)
www.aad.org

Allergies & Asthma

"Treat your symptoms before they get out of control. Don't feel too proud to get treatment. Know your limits! Remember to follow all of your doctor's instructions and don't be afraid to ask questions."

Dave S., University of Michigan

Allergies and asthma can be triggered by the same substances, but they are two different conditions.

With an **allergy**, the immune system reacts to a substance (allergen) that is normally harmless. An allergen can be inhaled, swallowed, or come in contact with the skin. Allergies refer to *many* conditions, such as eczema, hay fever, and a serious condition called anaphylaxis. This sudden, severe allergic reaction occurs within minutes of exposure. It is a medical emergency.

Asthma is *one* condition – a chronic, lower respiratory disease that affects the bronchial tubes (the main air passages in the lungs).

A person can have allergies without asthma; asthma with few or no allergies; or both. About 80% of asthma in children and about half of asthma in adults may be related to allergies.

Signs & Symptoms

For Common Allergies

- Runny, stuffy, or itchy nose. Sneezing. Burning, itchy, or watery eyes. Dark circles under the eyes.
- Itchy, irritated, or red skin (e.g., skin rash).
- Loss of smell or taste. Frequent throat clearing. Hoarseness. Coughing or wheezing.
- Repeated ear and sinus infections.

For a Severe Allergic Reaction

- Shortness of breath. A hard time breathing or swallowing. Wheezing.
- Severe swelling all over or of the face, lips, tongue, and/or throat.
- Pale or bluish lips, skin, and/or fingernails.
- Cool, moist skin or sudden onset of pale skin and sweating.
- Feeling dizzy, weak, and/or numb. Fainting. Decreasing level of awareness.

For Asthma

- A cough lasts more than a week. Coughing may be the only symptom. It may occur during the night or after exercising.
- Wheezing.
- Prolonged shortness of breath. Breathing gets harder and may hurt. It is harder to breathe out than in.
- Chest tightness or pain.

Causes & Risk Factors

In both allergies and asthma, the immune system releases chemicals that cause swelling. With asthma, the swelling is in the breathing tubes. With allergies, the inflammatory response can affect the eyes, nasal passages, the skin, etc.

For Allergies

- Breathing allergens from animal dander, dust, grass, weed and tree pollen, mold spores, etc.
- Ingesting allergens (e.g., food and medicines). Common food allergens are milk, fish, nuts, wheat, corn, and eggs. Common medicine allergens are penicillin and aspirin.

Common Health Problems

Allergies & Asthma, *Continued*

- Allergens that come in contact with the skin. Examples are cosmetics, latex, poison ivy, and metals. These can result in skin rashes like eczema, contact dermatitis, and hives.

{*Note:* Insect stings, nuts, penicillin, and shellfish are common causes of a severe allergic reaction.}

For Asthma

The exact cause for asthma is not known. A family history of it and/or having allergies increases the risk for asthma. It is also more common in children who live in houses with pets and/or tobacco smoke.

Asthma Attack Triggers

- Breathing an allergen (e.g., pollen, dust, mold, dander, etc.) or an irritant (e.g., tobacco smoke, air pollution, fumes, perfumes, etc.).
- Colds, flu, bronchitis, and sinus infections.
- Sulfites (additives in wine and some foods).
- Cold air. Temperature and humidity changes.
- Exercise, especially outdoors in cold air.
- Some medicines, such as aspirin.
- Strong feelings, including laughing and crying.
- Hormone changes with menstrual periods, etc.

Treatment

For Allergies

Avoid the allergen(s). Skin tests can identify allergens. Allergy shots may be prescribed. Medications can prevent and relieve symptoms. Medicine (e.g., an EpiPen), can be prescribed to use for a severe reaction before emergency care is given.

For Asthma

Asthma is too complex to treat with over-the-counter products. A doctor should diagnose and monitor asthma. He or she may prescribe one or more medicines. Some kinds are to be taken with an asthma attack. Other kinds are taken daily (or as prescribed) to help prevent asthma attacks.

A yearly flu vaccine is advised. Regular doctor visits are needed to detect any problems and evaluate your use of medicines.

Questions to Ask

Do any of these signs occur?
- Signs of a **severe allergic reaction** listed on page 12.
- Chest pain or tightening.
- Seizure.
- Cough that doesn't let up and a hard time breathing.

YES Get Immediate Care

NO

Do any of these signs occur?
- You can't say 4 or 5 words between breaths or eat or sleep due to shortness of breath.
- Wheezing and you are taking corticosteroid medicine.
- Wheezing doesn't stop after your prescribed treatment.
- A fever and heavy breathing.
- Your peak expiratory flow (PEF) reading on your peak flow meter is below 50% of your personal best number.

YES Get Immediate Care

NO

Flowchart continued on next page

Allergies & Asthma, *Continued*

Flowchart continued

Do any of these signs occur?
• Flushing, redness all over the body, or severe hives.
• Hoarseness.
• Anxiety. Trembling.
• Enlarged pupils.
• A severe reaction occurred in the past after exposure to a like substance.

YES Get Immediate Care

NO

Is your peak expiratory flow (PEF) 50 to 80% of your personal best number?

YES See Provider

NO

With asthma, do you have any of these problems?
• An asthma attack does not respond to self-care or prescribed medicine.
• Asthma attacks are coming more often and/or are getting worse.
• You use your bronchodilator more than 2 times a week.
• A cough keeps you awake at night.
• Signs of an infection occur, such as a fever and/or a cough with mucus that is green, yellow, or bloody-colored.

YES See Provider

NO

 Use Self-Care

See Self-Care in next column

Self-Care

For a Severe Allergic Reaction

■ Use prescribed medicine, such as an EpiPen, as advised. Then get emergency care!

■ Wear a medical ID alert tag for things that cause a severe allergic reaction.

■ Avoid things you are allergic to.

For Other Allergic Reactions

■ For hives and itching, take an OTC antihistamine, such as Benadryl. Take it as prescribed by your doctor or as directed on the label. {*Note:* If you have asthma, do not take an antihistamine.}

■ Don't use **hot** water for baths, showers, or to wash rash areas.

■ For itching, use an oatmeal bath or calamine (not Caladryl) lotion. Or, use a paste made with 3 tsp. of baking soda and 1 teaspoon of water.

■ Avoid things you are allergic to.

For Asthma

■ Don't smoke or let others smoke in your home. Stay away from smoke and air pollution.

■ Drink lots of liquids (2 to 3 quarts a day).

■ Wear a scarf around your mouth and nose when you are outside in cold weather to warm the air as you breathe it in. This prevents cold air from reaching sensitive airways.

■ Stop exercising if you start to wheeze.

■ Avoid your asthma triggers.

Allergies & Asthma, *Continued*

- Try to keep your dorm room or bedroom allergen-free.

  - Sleep with no pillow or the kind your doctor suggests. Use a plastic or "allergen-free" cover on your mattress and pillow (if you use one). Wash mattress pads in hot water every week.

  - Use curtains and throw rugs that can be washed often. Don't use drapes.

  - If you can, use a vacuum with a HEPA filter and double-thickness bags. Vacuum and dust often. Wear a dust filter mask when you do.

  - Reduce clutter in your room. Store items in plastic containers with lids.

  - Use a portable air purifier, such as one with a HEPA filter. In the summer, use an air conditioner, if possible.

- Don't consume things with sulfites, such as wine and some shellfish.

- Use your peak flow meter, as advised, to monitor your asthma.

- Sit up during an asthma attack.

- Keep your asthma rescue medicine handy. Take it as prescribed. Don't take over-the-counter medicines unless cleared first with your health care provider.

For Information, Contact:

Asthma and Allergy Foundation of America
800.7.ASTHMA (727.8462)
www.aafa.org

Colds & Flu

"I used to get colds often, especially around exam times. Now I make sure I wash my hands a lot. I think this helps me get fewer colds."

Sylvia P., Brooklyn College

Colds and seasonal flu are the main reason students miss class due to illness. Both are caused by viruses. Flu is short for influenza, a virus that affects your upper respiratory system. "Stomach flu" is stomach pain, diarrhea, vomiting, etc. caused by a virus in the stomach and intestines. For these symptoms, see "**Abdominal Pain**" on page 6, "**Diarrhea**" on page 23, and/or "**Vomiting & Nausea**" on page 64.

Is it a cold or is it the flu? See the chart on page 16 that compares their signs and symptoms.

Flu symptoms come on suddenly and affect the body all over. Cold symptoms mostly affect you above the neck. When you get the flu, you are more prone to bronchitis and sinus and ear infections.

Prevention

- Wash your hands often with soap and water. Keep them away from your nose, eyes, and mouth. Use an instant hand sanitizer when you can't wash your hands.

- Try to avoid close contact with people and their things when they have a cold or the flu.

- Cover your nose and mouth with a tissue when you cough or sneeze. Throw the tissue away after you use it.

- Get a yearly seasonal flu vaccine and other flu vaccines as advised.

Common Health Problems

Common Health Problems

Colds & Flu, *Continued*

Signs & Symptoms

Colds & Flu Comparison Chart			
Signs & Symptoms	**Cold**	**Flu**	**H1N1 Flu**
Fever / Chills	Rare / not common	Common. Can be high fever.	Usual. 20% of people may not have a fever.
Headache	Not common	Common	Very common
Body Aches	Slight	Severe	Severe
Runny, stuffy nose	Common	Runny nose is common	Not common
Sneezing	Common	Common	Not common
Sore throat	Common	Common	Not common
Cough	Cough with mucus	Often. Dry and hacking cough.	Usual. Dry cough without mucus.
Diarrhea / Vomiting	None	Not common. More likely to occur in children than adults.	Sometimes
Chest discomfort	Mild to moderate	Moderate	Often severe

Other Forms of Flu

Bird flu. This is caused by avian influenza viruses which normally infect wild birds. Contact with infected birds or surfaces they contaminate can spread these viruses to humans. The viruses may be able to change to a form that could spread from person-to-person and result in a widespread infection in humans.

Pandemic flu. This is a term for any type of flu that causes a global outbreak of serious illness that spreads easily from person-to-person.

Treatment

Self-care (see page 18) treats colds and most cases of the flu.

Prescribed antiviral medicines may make flu symptoms milder and help you recover sooner if started within 48 hours of the onset of flu symptoms. Antibiotics **do not** treat cold and flu viruses.

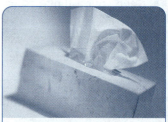

Prevent spreading cold and flu viruses. Use tissues when you blow your nose.

Colds & Flu, *Continued*

Questions to Ask

With or following the flu, do any of the following **symptoms of meningitis** occur?
- Stiff neck (can't bend the head forward to touch the chin to the chest).
- Severe headache that persists.
- Red or purple rash that doesn't fade after the skin is pressed.
- Seizure.
- Lethargy.

YES → Get Immediate Care

NO ↓

After a recent case of the flu, are any of these **signs of Reye's Syndrome** present?
- Sudden, repeated vomiting.
- Pain in the upper right area of the abdomen.
- Rapid mental status changes (agitation, confusion, delirium).
- Increased pulse and breathing rate.
- Lethargy.
- Decreasing level of awareness.

YES → Get Immediate Care

NO ↓

With the flu, do you have severe or increasing shortness of breath or severe wheezing?

YES → Get Immediate Care

NO ↓

Flowchart continued in next column

Do you have 2 or more of these **signs and symptoms of a sinus infection**?
- Fever over 101°F (38.3°C).
- Green, yellow, or bloody-colored nasal discharge for more than 3 days. A drainage into the back of the throat that tastes bad may occur.
- Pain (usually throbbing) around the eye(s), cheek(s), upper jaw(s), and/or between the nose and eye socket(s).
- Headache worsens when you bend forward. OTC pain relievers don't stop the pain.

YES → See Provider

NO ↓

With a cold or flu do you have any of these problems?
- A fever over 104°F (40°C).
- A sore throat that is bright red or has white spots.
- An earache that persists.
- A cough with mucus that is yellow, green, or gray.
- Fever or other symptoms like coughing are getting worse.

YES → See Provider

NO ↓

Have you had a cold or the flu for more than a week and not felt better using Self-Care? Or, do you have new symptoms?

YES → Call Provider

NO ↓

 Use Self-Care

Common Health Problems

Colds & Flu, *Continued*

Self-Care

■ Drink lots of liquids.

■ Take an over-the-counter medicine for muscle aches, and/or fever, but don't take aspirin if you have flu-like symptoms. (See "**Pain Relievers**" in "**Over-the-Counter Medication Safety**" on page 75.)

■ Use an over-the-counter saline nasal spray, such as Ocean brand. Use as directed on the label.

■ Use a cool-mist vaporizer in your room.

■ Have chicken soup. It helps clear mucus.

■ Take echinacea, zinc lozenges, and/or vitamin C, as advised by your health care provider, when cold or flu symptoms start. Don't take echinacea and/or zinc lozenges long term. These do not prevent colds and flu.

For a Sore Throat

■ Gargle every few hours with a solution of ¹/₄ teaspoon of salt dissolved in 1 cup of warm water. Make sure the salt is dissolved.

■ Drink tea with lemon (with or without honey).

■ Suck on hard candy or a medicated lozenge.

■ See, also, **"To Treat a Sore Throat"** on page 44.

For Information, Contact:

The Centers for Disease Control and Prevention
800.CDC.INFO (232.4636)
www.flu.gov and www.cdc.gov/flu

Coughs

"The air in the dorm is so dry, that it makes a lot of us cough at night. We find that a cheap humidifier or even a large bowl of water in the room adds enough moisture to relieve those nightly coughs."

Rachael G., Cornell University

Coughing clears the lungs and airways. Coughing is only a symptom, not the problem.

Signs & Symptoms

There are 3 kinds of coughs:

■ Productive. This brings up mucus or phlegm.

■ Nonproductive. This is a dry cough.

■ Reflex. This is a cough that comes from a problem somewhere else, like the ear or stomach.

Causes

■ Tobacco smoke.

■ Dry air.

■ Infections. Examples are bronchitis, colds, and the flu. (See "**Colds & Flu**" on page 15.)

■ Allergies and postnasal drip.

■ Asthma.

Other causes include having something stuck in your windpipe and acid reflux from the stomach that comes with heartburn. Coughing can also be a symptom of a medical condition, such as asthma.

Coughs, *Continued*

Treatment

How to treat your cough depends on what kind it is. Treat the cause and soothe the irritation. Stay away from smoking and secondhand smoke. Smoke hurts your lungs and makes it harder for your body to fight an infection.

Questions to Ask

With coughing, do you have signs of a **severe allergic reaction**?
- A hard time breathing or swallowing.
- Severe swelling all over, or of the face, lips, tongue, and/or throat.
- Obstructed airway.
- Wheezing.
- Dizziness, weakness.

YES → Get Immediate Care

NO

With a cough, do you have any of these problems?
- A hard time breathing.
- Fainting.
- You cough up true red blood.

YES → Get Immediate Care

NO

Does a cough persist after an episode of choking on food or a foreign object?

YES → Get Immediate Care

NO

Flowchart continued in next column

With a cough, do you have any of these problems?
- An itchy, red splotchy rash.
- A fever of 102°F (38.8°C) or higher.
- Your chest hurts only when you cough and the pain goes away when you sit up or lean forward.
- You cough up green, yellow, or bloody-colored mucus.
- You lose weight for no reason, have fatigue, and sweat a lot at night.

YES → See Provider

NO

Does your cough last for more than 2 weeks without getting better?

YES → Call Provider

NO

 Use Self-Care

Self-Care

For Coughs that Bring Up Mucus

- Drink plenty of liquids, such as water, hot tea, and fruit juice.

- Use a cool-mist vaporizer in your room.

- Take a shower. The steam helps thin mucus.

- Take an over-the-counter expectorant or cough medicine with guaifenesin. Take it as directed.

- Don't smoke. Avoid secondhand smoke.

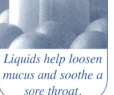

Liquids help loosen mucus and soothe a sore throat.

Coughs, *Continued*

For Coughs that Are Dry

- Drink liquids. Have warm tea, chicken soup, etc.
- Suck on cough drops or hard candy.
- Take an over-the-counter cough medicine that contains dextromethorphan. Take it as directed.

Depression

"Feeling depressed is so common among girls in my dorm that I thought it was just a normal part of college. When it got to be too much for me to handle, I went to the Counseling Center. With the counselor's help, I'm coping with my moods much better now."

Mary L., University of Cincinnati

Depression is the most common reason college students go to their school's counseling service. Depression makes a person less able to manage life. It affects a person's mood, mind, body, and behaviors.

Signs & Symptoms

A person who is depressed has one or more of the signs and symptoms listed below.

- Feeling sad, hopeless, and helpless.
- Feeling guilty and/or worthless.
- Thinking negative thoughts.
- Having a loss of interest in things, such as social activities, hobbies, and sex.
- Sleeping too little or too much.
- Fatigue or loss of energy.
- Problems concentrating or making decisions.
- Ongoing physical symptoms, such as headaches, chronic pain, or digestive problems that don't respond to treatment.
- Uncontrollable crying.
- Poor appetite with weight loss, or overeating and weight gain.
- Thoughts of suicide or death.

The number and severity of the symptoms vary from person to person.

Causes & Risk Factors

- Major changes and stress that accompany college, including choosing career goals, leaving home, and the strain from trying to study and socialize at the same time.
- Obsessing about expenses.
- Abuse of alcohol, drugs, and some medications.
- Relationship changes, such as break ups, a family divorce, or the death of someone close.
- Brain chemical imbalances. Also, some types of depression run in families.
- Hormonal changes. This could be from taking birth control pills or using anabolic steroids which can cause changes in mood.
- Lack of natural, unfiltered sunlight between late fall and spring. This is called Seasonal Affective Disorder (SAD). It may only affect some people that are prone to this disorder.
- Holiday "blues."

Depression, *Continued*

Most likely, depression is caused by a mix of: A family history of the illness; brain chemical imbalances; emotional issues; and other factors, such as a medical illness or alcohol abuse.

In some people, events like extreme stress and grief may cause depression. In others, depression occurs even when life is going well.

Treatment

Treatment includes medicines, psychotherapy, and other therapies that are specific to the cause of the depression. Exposure to bright lights (similar to sunlight) for depression that results from SAD can be helpful. {*Note:* Some antidepressant medicines can increase the risk for suicidal thoughts and behaviors, especially in children and adolescents. This risk may be higher within the first days to a month after starting the medicine. Persons who take antidepressants should be closely monitored.}

Questions to Ask

Have you just attempted suicide, written a suicide note, or are you planning suicide? Do you have persistent thoughts of suicide or death? **YES** Get Immediate Care

NO

Have you had a lot less interest or pleasure in almost all activities most of the day, nearly every day for at least 2 weeks? **YES** See Provider

NO

Flowchart continued in next column

Have you been depressed most of the day, nearly every day <u>and</u> had any of these problems for at least 2 weeks?
• Feeling hopeless, worthless, guilty, slowed down, or restless.
• Changes in appetite or weight.
• Thoughts of death or suicide.
• Problems concentrating, thinking, remembering, or making decisions.
• Trouble sleeping or sleeping too much.
• Feeling tired all of the time.
• Headaches or other aches and pains.
• Digestive problems.
• Sexual problems.
• Feeling anxious or worried.

YES See Provider

NO

Has depression kept you from doing daily tasks for more than 2 weeks and caused you to withdraw from normal activities? **YES** See Provider

NO

Has the depression occurred as the result of any of the following?
• Taking over-the-counter or a prescribed medication.
• Abusing alcohol or drugs.
• A medical problem.
• Recent delivery of a baby.

YES Call Provider

NO

Flowchart continued on next page

 To Learn More, See Back Cover

Depression, *Continued*

Flowchart continued

Are you feeling depressed now and do any of the following apply?
- You have been depressed before and not received treatment or you have been treated for depression in the past and it has returned.
- You have taken medication for depression in the past.
- A close relative has a history of depression.

YES → **See Provider**

NO ↓

During holiday times, do you withdraw from family and friends and/or dwell on past holidays to the point that it interferes with your present life?

YES → **Call Provider**

NO ↓

Does the depression come with dark, cloudy weather or winter months and does it lift when spring comes?

YES → **Call Provider**

NO ↓

 Use Self-Care

Self-Care

■ Take medications as prescribed. Get your doctor's advice before you take over-the-counter herbs, such as St. John's Wort, especially if you take other medications.

■ Don't use illegal drugs. Limit alcohol. These can cause or worsen depression. Drugs and alcohol can also make medicines for depression less effective. Harmful side effects can occur when drugs and/or alcohol are mixed with medicine.

■ Eat healthy foods. Eat at regular times.

■ Get regular exercise.

■ Talk to someone who will listen to the tensions and frustrations you are feeling.

■ Try not to isolate yourself. Be with people you trust and feel safe with, even though you feel down.

■ Do things you enjoy. Do something that lets you express yourself. Draw. Paint. Write your thoughts in a diary or journal.

■ Relax. Listen to soft music, take a warm bath or shower. Do relaxation exercises.

■ Avoid stressful situations or taking on added commitments when you feel depressed.

■ Keep an emergency number handy (e.g., crisis hotline, trusted friend's number, etc.) in case you feel desperate.

Feeling better takes time. Don't expect to just "snap out" of your depression.

To Help A Friend Who Is Depressed

■ Help your friend get an appropriate diagnosis. Make an initial appointment with a professional and offer to take your friend.

■ Do not ignore remarks about suicide. Report them, immediately, to a student advisor, teacher, or health care provider.

Depression, *Continued*

- Be aware of the type of medication your friend needs to take and when it should be taken. If necessary, alert your friend's health care provider about any side effects that you notice.

- Be supportive. Depression is no different from any other physical illness. It requires patience, understanding, love, and encouragement. Encourage your friend to continue with treatment and to see his or her health care provider if there is no improvement.

- Listen with care. Point out your friend's successes and attributes when he or she feels worthless, helpless, or down about the future. Helping your friend see previous successes can help give the confidence needed to continue with treatment. Your friend doesn't need you to tell him or her what to do. Listening is very helpful.

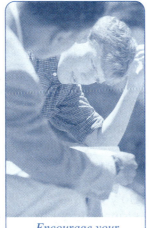

Encourage your friend to talk about his or her feelings.

- Encourage your friend to go out and do things with you or with others, such as to see a movie or to do things your friend enjoyed in the past. Don't push, though, or make too many demands.

- Seek support from organizations (see places listed in the next column) that deal with depression.

For Information, Contact:

Your school's Student Counseling Service or Student Mental Health Service.
(Normally, these services are no cost to you.)

International Foundation for Research and Education on Depression (IFRED)
www.ifred.org

Mental Health America (MHA)
800.969.6642 • www.mentalhealthamerica.net

National Mental Health Consumers' Self-Help Clearinghouse
800.553.4539 • www.mhselfhelp.org

Diarrhea

"My first night in the dorm, I was nervous with an upset stomach. The fact that I had to use a community bathroom made it even more uncomfortable."

Susan S., Rutgers University

Diarrhea is passing body waste from the bowel more often and in a more liquid state than usual.

Signs & Symptoms

- Frequent watery, loose stools.
- Cramping or pain in the abdomen.

Common Health Problems

Diarrhea, *Continued*

Causes

- "Stomach flu," which is a viral infection of the intestines.
- Spoiled food, contaminated water, or infections from bacteria or parasites that affect the digestive tract. One example is traveler's diarrhea.
- Overuse of alcohol or laxatives.
- A side effect of some medicines, such as some antibiotics.
- Lactose intolerance or a food allergy.
- Menstrual cramps.
- Stress or a panic attack.

Diarrhea is also a symptom of health conditions, such as irritable bowel syndrome ("spastic colon"). It results in irregular bowel habits and abdominal pain that are not due to any other bowel disease.

Prevention

- Wash your hands after going to the toilet and before preparing food. Use disposable paper towels to dry your hands.
- When traveling, find out if it is advisable to drink bottled water, boiled water, and to avoid using ice cubes. You may need to remove the peels from fruits and vegetables before eating.

Treatment

Self-care treats most bouts of diarrhea. If the diarrhea is caused by a medical condition, treating it will help alleviate the diarrhea.

Questions to Ask

With diarrhea, do you have these **signs of dehydration**?
- Sunken and dry or tearless eyes.
- Dry mouth, tongue, and lips.
- No urine or a low amount of urine that is dark yellow.
- Lightheadedness, especially when getting up quickly.
- Dry skin that doesn't spring back after being pinched.
- Dizziness, confusion, weakness.
- Increase in breathing and heart rate.
- Severe thirst (sometimes).

YES → Get Immediate Care

NO ↓

Is there blood in the diarrhea or is its color tarlike or maroon? **YES** → Get Immediate Care

NO ↓

Do you have the following **signs and symptoms of irritable bowel syndrome**?
- Gas, bloating, cramps, or pain in the abdomen.
- Changes in bowel habits:
  - Constipation, diarrhea, or both.
  - Crampy urge, but inability to move your bowels.
  - Mucus in your stool.

YES →   See Provider

NO ↓

Flowchart continued on next page

Diarrhea, *Continued*

Flowchart continued

Do you have any of these problems with diarrhea?
- Temperature of 101°F (38.3°C) or higher.
- The diarrhea has lasted for 48 hours or longer.
- You have a chronic illness and have diarrhea more than 8 times a day.
- You are taking medicines (regular medicines that the body may not be absorbing due to the diarrhea, and/or prescribed or over-the-counter ones that might be contributing to the diarrhea).

YES Call Provider

NO

Did diarrhea occur on, during, or after returning from a foreign country?

YES Call Provider

NO

 Use Self-Care

Self-Care

- If vomiting is also present, treat for vomiting first. (See "**Vomiting & Nausea**" topic on page 64.)

- Follow your normal diet if there are no **signs of dehydration** (see previous page).

- Until the diarrhea subsides, avoid caffeine, milk products, and foods that are greasy, high in fiber, or very sweet.

- If there are **signs of dehydration**, stop solid foods. Have around 2 cups of clear fluids per hour (if vomiting isn't present). Fluids of choice are:
  - Sport drinks, such as Gatorade.
  - Kool-Aid. This usually has less sugar than soda pop.

- Don't drink just clear liquids for more than 24 hours.

- Avoid having high "simple" sugar drinks, like apple juice, grape juice, gelatin, regular colas, and other soft drinks. These can pull water into the gut and make the diarrhea persist.

- Start eating normal meals within 12 hours. Good food choices are:
  - Starchy foods, such as rice, potatoes, cereals (not sweetened ones), crackers, and toast.
  - Vegetables, such as cooked carrots, and non milk-based soups with noodles, rice, and/or vegetables.
  - Lean (not fatty) meats.
  - Yogurt, especially with live active cultures of lactobacillus acidophilus.

- Use over-the-counter lactobacillus acidophilus capsules or tablets. These help restore normal bacteria to the bowel.

- Avoid fatty and fried foods.

- The B.R.A.T. diet: Just having bananas, rice, applesauce, and dry toast is no longer the diet of choice for diarrhea. These foods are still okay to eat, though.

- Exercise moderately until the diarrhea is gone.

- Try an over-the-counter antidiarrheal medicine, such as Imodium A-D, but wait at least 12 hours before you take this to let the diarrhea "run its course" to get rid of what caused it.

Diarrhea, *Continued*

For Lactose Intolerance

- Avoid foods that are not easy for you to digest. Some people with lactose intolerance can tolerate dairy products in small portions.

- Try foods that have had lactose reduced by bacterial cultures. Examples are buttermilk, yogurt, and sweet acidophilus milk. Take over-the-counter lactobacillus acidophilus capsules.

- Take over-the-counter drops or pills that have the enzyme lactase when you have dairy foods.

- If the above measures don't help, avoid products with milk, milk solids, and whey. Products marked "parve" are milk free.

Eating Disorders

"One night, I sat and watched my roommate enjoy eating a bagel with cream cheese and drinking hot chocolate. I wish I could enjoy food that much. I take hours contemplating calories before I can put anything in my mouth."

Angelina R., University of Texas

Five to 10 million adolescent girls and women have an eating disorder. About 1 million males do. The 3 most common eating disorders are anorexia nervosa, bulimia nervosa, and binge eating disorder. These eating disorders are a coping mechanism. They result in an obsession with food and/or weight; anxiety around eating; guilt; and severe and adverse effects on psychological and physical health. Eating disorders are very serious health problems.

Signs & Symptoms

For Anorexia Nervosa

- Loss of a lot of weight in a short period of time.

- Intense, irrational fear of weight gain and/or of looking fat. Obsession with fat, calories, and weight.

- Distorted body image. Despite being below a normal weight for height and age, the person feels and sees himself or herself as fat.

- A need to be perfect or in control in one area of life.

- Marked physical signs. These include loss of hair, slowed heart rate, low blood pressure, and feeling cold due to decrease in body temperature. In females, menstrual periods can stop.

For Bulimia Nervosa

- Repeated acts of binge eating and purging. Purging can be through vomiting; taking laxatives, water pills, and/or diet pills; fasting; and exercising excessively to "undo" the binge.

- Excessive concern about body weight.

- Being overweight, underweight, or normal weight.

- Dieting often.

- Dental problems, mouth sores, and a chronic sore throat.

- Spending a lot of time in bathrooms.

- Because of binge-purge cycles, severe health problems can occur. These include an irregular heartbeat and damage to the stomach, kidneys, and bones.

Eating Disorders, *Continued*

For Binge Eating Disorder

- Periods of nonstop eating that are unrelated to hunger.

- Impulsive binging on food without purging.

- Repeated use of diets or sporadic fasts.

- Weight can range from normal weight to mild, moderate, or severe obesity.

Causes & Risk Factors

An exact cause has not been found. Persons from all backgrounds, ages, genders, and ethnic cultures are affected. Risk factors include:

- A family history of eating disorders.

- Pressure from society to be thin.

- Personal and family pressures.

- A history of sexual, physical, or alcohol abuse.

- Fear of starting puberty or of sexual relations.

- Pressure for athletes to lose weight (sometimes quickly to qualify for an event) or to be thin for competitive sports.

- Chronic dieting.

Treatment

The earlier the condition is diagnosed and treated, the better the outcome. Treatment includes:

- Counseling. This can be in individual, family, group, and/or behavioral therapy.

- Support groups.

- Medication.

- Nutrition therapy.

- Outpatient treatment or hospitalization.

Questions to Ask

Are you thinking about or making plans for suicide? **YES** → **Get Immediate Care**

NO

Did you binge and purge, fast, diet, and/or exercise on purpose to lose more than 10 pounds <u>and</u> do you have any of these problems?
- An intense fear of gaining weight or of getting fat.
- You see yourself as fat even though you are at normal weight or are underweight.
- You diet and exercise in excess after reaching your goal weight.

YES → **See Provider**

NO

Do you have episodes of eating a large amount of food within 2 hours and can't control the amount of food you eat or can't stop eating? And, do you do at least 3 of these things?
- Eat very fast.
- Eat until you feel uncomfortable.
- Eat when you are not hungry.
- Eat alone due to embarrassment.
- Feel depressed, disgusted, and/or guilty after you overeat.

YES → **See Provider**

NO

Flowchart continued on next page

Common Health Problems

Eating Disorders, *Continued*

Flowchart continued

Do you hoard food, induce vomiting, and/or spend a lot of time in the bathroom from taking laxatives or water pills? **YES** → **See Provider**

NO ↓

With abnormal eating, do you have 2 or more of these problems?
• Rapid tooth decay.
• Low body temperature. Cold hands and feet.
• Thin hair (or hair loss) on the head. Baby-like hair growth on the body.
• Problems with digestion. Bloating. Constipation.
• Three or more missed periods in a row or delayed onset of menstruation.
• Times when you are depressed, euphoric, and/or hyperactive.
• Tiredness or tremors.
• Lack of concentration.

YES → **See Provider**

NO ↓

 Use Self-Care

Self-Care

Eating disorders need professional help.

To Help Prevent an Eating Disorder

■ Learn to accept yourself and your body. You don't need to be or look like anyone else. Spend time 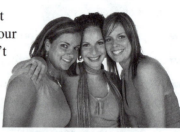 with people who accept you as you are, not people who focus on "thinness."

■ Know that self-esteem does not have to depend on body weight.

■ Eat nutritious foods. Focus on whole grains, beans, fresh fruits and vegetables, low-fat dairy foods, and lean meats.

■ Commit to a goal of normal eating. Realize that this will take time. It will also take courage to fight fears of gaining weight.

■ Don't skip meals. If you do, you are more likely to binge when you eat.

■ Avoid white flour, sugar and foods high in sugar and fat, such as cakes, cookies, and pastries. Bulimics tend to binge on junk food. The more they eat, the more they want.

■ Get regular moderate exercise 3 to 4 times a week. If you exercise more than your doctor advises, do non-exercise activities with friends and family.

Eating Disorders, *Continued*

- Find success in things that you do. Hobbies, work, school, etc. can promote self-esteem.

- Learn as much as you can about eating disorders from books and places that deal with them.

- To help their children avoid eating disorders, parents should promote a balance between their child's competing needs for independence and family involvement.

If You Have an Eating Disorder

- Follow your treatment plan.

- Attend counseling sessions and/or support group meetings as scheduled.

- Identify feelings before, during, and after you overeat, binge, purge, or restrict food intake. What is it that you are hoping the food will do?

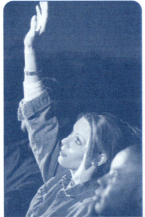

Support groups can be very helpful for persons with an eating disorder.

- Set small goals that you can easily reach. Congratulate yourself for every success. This is a process. Accept setbacks. Learn from them.

- Talk to someone instead of turning to food.

- Learn to recognize your personal rights and to state how you feel. You have the right to say no and the right to express your feelings and your opinions. You have the right to ask that your needs are met.

- Keep a journal of your progress, feelings, and thoughts, but not about what you eat. The journal is just for you, not for others to read or judge. This is a safe place to be honest with yourself. The journal can also help you identify your "triggers" so that you can deal with them in the future.

- Don't let the scale run your life. Better yet, throw out the scale!

For Information, Contact:

Your school's Student Health Service, Student Counseling or Mental Health Service

National Eating Disorders Association Information and Referral Helpline
800.931.2237
www.nationaleatingdisorders.org

Something Fishy Website on Eating Disorders
866.690.7239
www.something-fishy.org

Fatigue

"I read on a bulletin board that the average college student, left in a dark room, will fall asleep within 10 minutes. I bet I could beat that time by half!"

Mark E., Syracuse University

Being tired due to a busy schedule and lack of sleep is normal. Being fatigued, on the other hand, could be a symptom of a health condition.

Signs & Symptoms

Fatigue is being more than tired. With fatigue, you:

- Feel drained of energy and have a very hard time doing normal activities and school work.
- Have low motivation and may miss classes often.
- Feel inadequate and have little desire for sex.

Causes

- Lack of sleep for long periods of time.
- Burnout and stress.
- Crash dieting and eating poorly.
- Side effects from allergies.

Health conditions that lead to fatigue include:

- Alcohol or drug abuse.
- Anemia.
- Autoimmune disorders, including thyroid disease, diabetes, and lupus (the systemic type).
- Chronic fatigue syndrome. The fatigue lasts at least 6 months.
- Depression.
- Hepatitis.
- HIV/AIDS (see page 49).

Mononucleosis ("Mono")

A common cause of fatigue in students is **infectious mononucleosis**, an acute viral disease.

Signs & Symptoms

- Fatigue.
- Fever.
- Sore throat.
- Swollen lymph gland in the neck area.
- Pain in the upper left abdominal area.

Symptoms usually last several weeks.

Cause

Epstein-Barr virus (EBV). This is spread from person to person through contact with saliva from a person recently infected with the disease. The saliva can be picked up from hand-to-hand contact, sharing eating utensils, and kissing, which is why "Mono" is called the "kissing disease." Symptoms usually appear about 4 to 6 weeks after exposure.

Treatment

Rest is the mainstay of treatment. Avoiding heavy lifting and contact sports is necessary, because there is a risk of rupturing the spleen with "Mono."

Questions to Ask

With debilitating fatigue, do you have **signs and symptoms of infectious mononucleosis** listed above?

YES See Provider

NO

Flowchart continued on next page

30

Fatigue, *Continued*

Flowchart continued

With fatigue, do you also have these **signs and symptoms of hepatitis**?
- The whites of your eyes and/or skin looks yellow (jaundice).
- Dark-colored urine.
- Vomiting and nausea.
- Loss of weight or appetite.
- Pain in the abdomen.
- Fever.
- Stools are pale and clay-colored.

{**Note:** With some forms of hepatitis, no symptoms are present.}

YES See Provider

NO

With fatigue and weakness, do you have any of the following **signs of diabetes**?
- Constant urination.
- Abnormally increased thirst and increased hunger.
- Rapid weight loss or excessive weight gain.
- Extreme irritability.
- Nausea and vomiting.
- Drowsiness.
- Itching and/or skin infections that don't clear up easily.
- Tingling, numbness, or pain in the arms and legs.
- Blurred vision.

YES See Provider

NO

Flowchart continued in next column

With fatigue, do you have **signs and symptoms of hypothyroidism**?
- Hair loss and dry, thick, flaky skin.
- Decreased tolerance to cold temperatures and numbness or tingling in the hands.
- Unexplained weight gain.
- Constipation.
- Sleepiness; feeling mentally sluggish.
- For females, longer and heavier menstrual periods.

YES 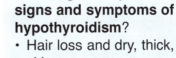 See Provider

NO

With fatigue, do you have other **signs and symptoms of multiple sclerosis**?
- Blurred vision, double vision, or the loss of vision in one eye.
- Bladder problems (frequent urination, urgency, infection, as well as incontinence).
- Feelings of pins and needles in the limbs.
- Muscle spasms.
- Leg stiffness. Unsteady gait.
- Poor coordination.
- Emotional mood swings, irritability, depression, anxiety, euphoria.

YES See Provider

NO

Flowchart continued on next page

Fatigue, *Continued*

Flowchart continued

With fatigue, do you have any of these **signs and symptoms of lupus**?

• Joint pain for more than 3 months.
• Fingers that get pale, numb, or uncomfortable in the cold.
• Mouth sores for more than 2 weeks.
• Low blood counts from anemia, low white-cell count, or low platelet count.
• A butterfly-shaped rash on your cheeks for more than 1 month.
• Skin rash (raised patches with scaling) after being in the sun.
• Pain for more than 2 days when taking deep breaths.

YES → 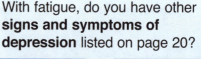 See Provider

NO ↓

With fatigue and weakness, do you have **signs and symptoms of anemia**?

• Shortness of breath with exertion.
• Paleness of the skin or paleness around the gums, nail beds, and/or linings of the lower eyelids.
• Headache.

YES → See Provider

NO ↓

Flowchart continued in next column

With fatigue, do you have other **signs and symptoms of depression** listed on page 20?

YES → See Provider

NO ↓

With debilitating fatigue, do you have **signs and symptoms of fibromyalgia**?

• Muscle pain for more than 2 weeks.
• Flu-like symptoms. (See **Signs & Symptoms** of the **Flu** listed on page 16.)
• Insomnia.
• Mental fogginess.
• Headache.

YES → See Provider

NO ↓

Are any of the following linked with the fatigue?

• It occurred for no apparent reason, lasted for more than 2 weeks, and has kept you from doing your usual activities.
• The fatigue started after taking medicine.
• For a female, the fatigue hits hard right before or after each monthly menstrual period.
• Pregnancy is a possibility.

YES → See Provider

NO ↓

With fatigue that comes on suddenly, do you have **Signs and Symptoms** of the **Flu** listed on page 16?

YES →   Call Provider

NO ↓

 Use Self-Care

Fatigue, *Continued*

Self-Care

- Be organized. Use a daily/weekly/monthly planner to keep abreast of everything you need to do. Prioritize daily tasks, semester goals, etc. Make sure to plan time for exercise, eating, recreation, and sleep. Contact your student Mental Health Service or your academic counselor if you need help or feel overwhelmed.

- Take only the number of semester credits you can handle.

- Don't overextend yourself in extracurricular activities.

- Eat well. Eating too much and "crash dieting" are both hard on your body. Don't skip breakfast. Limit high-fat and/or rich, sugary snacks. Eat whole-grain breads and cereals and raw fruits and vegetables. Keep healthy snacks or meal replacement bars in your backpack to eat when you don't have time to have a meal.

- Get regular physical exercise. Use your school's fitness facilities and/or participate in organized sports, etc.

- Do something for yourself. Do things that also meet your needs, not just those of others.

- Avoid too much caffeine and alcohol. Don't abuse drugs. Don't use over-the-counter diet pills and stay awake pills (e.g., No-Doz). Repeated use of these can make you anxious, jittery, and unable to sleep.

- If fatigue is due to a medical condition, follow your health care provider's guidelines regarding rest, diet, medication, etc.

- Set up good sleep habits (see page 87).

Fever

"My temperature was so high, I felt like a barbeque grill in the summertime. I was too sick to go to class. It was very frightening."

Robert S., NYU

When you don't feel well and call a health care provider, you will most likely be asked if you have a fever.

Keep a thermometer in your dorm room or

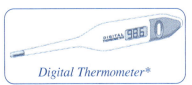

Digital Thermometer*

apartment to take your temperature when necessary. Use a digital one with disposable plastic probe covers. Use it as directed.

Glass mercury thermometers are not allowed in dorm rooms. If they break, droplets of toxic mercury can be released.

Signs & Symptoms

Normal body temperature is about 98.6°F (37°C). When you have a fever:

- Your temperature is higher than 99.5°F (37.5°C).

- Your skin feels warm.

Causes

Fever is one way the body fights an infection or illness. It helps speed up the body's defense actions by increasing blood flow.

Common Health Problems

Fever, *Continued*

Body temperature changes during the day. It is lowest in the morning and highest in the evening.

Other factors that can affect your temperature reading include wearing too much clothing, exercise, and hot, humid weather. Also, a female's hormones can cause her temperature to go up at certain times of the month, such as with ovulation.

Treatment

If having a fever up to 102°F (38.8°C) causes you no harm or discomfort and you have no other medical symptoms or medical problems, you may not need to treat it. If the fever makes you uncomfortable, is 102°F (38.8°C) or higher, if you have other symptoms and/or a medical condition, such as asthma, or if your fever lasts more than 3 days, you should seek medical care.

Questions to Ask

With a fever, do you have any of these problems?
- Seizure.
- Listlessness.
- Abnormal breathing.
- Stiff neck. (You can't touch your chin to your chest.)
- Excessive irritability.
- Confusion.
- Severe, persistent headache.

YES Get Immediate Care

NO

Is the fever 102°F (38.8°C) or higher for 36 or more hours?

YES See Provider

NO

Flowchart continued in next column

With a fever, do you have any of these problems?
- Persistent ear pain or pain in the sinuses (face).
- Persistent sore throat.
- Pain in the chest with deep breaths.
- Green, yellow, or bloody-colored discharge from the nose, throat, or ears.
- Urinary pain, burning, or frequency.
- Redness, swelling, and pain anywhere on the body.

YES 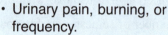 See Provider

NO

Has the fever done any of the following?
- Gone away for more than 24 hours and then come back.
- Comes soon after a visit to a foreign country.

YES Call Provider

NO

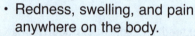 Use Self-Care

Self-Care

To Prevent a Fever

- Avoid very hot conditions.

- Drink plenty of fluids.

- To fight off infections, eat well, get plenty of rest, and exercise on a regular basis. Also, get recommended immunizations (see page 81).

Fever, *Continued*

To Treat a Fever

- Drink at least 1 to 2 quarts of liquids every day. This includes water, fruit juice, etc.

- Take a sponge bath with tepid (about 70°F; 21.1°C) water (not alcohol).

- Take the right dose of an over-the-counter medicine to reduce fever. (See "**Pain Relievers**" in "**Over-the-Counter Medication Safety**" on page 75.)

- Rest.

- Don't wear too many clothes or use too many blankets.

- Don't do heavy exercise.

Headaches

"It's tough to keep your face in a book for hours at a time. When I have a lot of reading to do, I take a 10 minute break for every hour I am studying to stop getting headaches."

Amy C., Michigan State University

Headaches are one of the most common health complaints, not just for college students, but for adults and even children.

Prevention

- Keep a diary of when, where, and why the headaches occur.

- Be aware of early symptoms. Try to stop the headache as soon as it begins.

- Exercise on a regular basis.

- Keep regular sleeping times, as much as you can.

- Don't smoke. If you smoke, quit. (See "**Tobacco Use – Benefits of Quitting**" on page 88.)

- Avoid excess alcohol.

Signs, Symptoms & Causes

Symptoms depend on the type of headache.

Tension or Muscular Headaches

Most headaches are this type. Signs and symptoms:

- A dull ache in your forehead, above your ears, or at the back of your head.

- Pain in your neck or shoulders that travels to your head.

Tension headaches are caused by tense or tight muscles in the face, neck, or scalp. You can get a tension headache from a number of things:

- Not getting enough sleep.

- Feeling "stressed out."

- Reading for long periods of time or eyestrain.

- Doing repetitive work.

- Staying in one position for a long time, such as working at a computer.

Migraine Headaches

Migraine headaches happen when blood vessels in your head open too wide or close too tight. Signs and symptoms:

- Headaches start on one side of your head. One side of your head hurts more than the other.

- Nausea or vomiting.

To Learn More, See Back Cover

Headaches, *Continued*

- Light hurts your eyes, noise bothers you. The headache is worse with activity.

- After the headache, some people have a drained feeling with tired, aching muscles. Others feel great after the headache goes away.

Migraines can occur with or without an aura. With an aura, spots or flashing lights or numbness occurs for 10 to 30 minutes before the headache. Ten percent of all migraines are this type; 90% occur without an aura.

Migraine headaches occur more often in females than in males and tend to run in families.

Certain things trigger migraine headaches in susceptible people. They include:

- Menstruation in females.

- Caffeine, alcohol, and/or certain foods, such as aged cheeses, cured meats (hot dogs, ham, etc.).

- Stress. Changes in sleeping patterns.

- Strenuous exercise.

Sinus Headaches

A sinus headache occurs when fluids in the nose aren't able to drain well and a buildup of pressure occurs in the sinuses. A cold, allergies, and airplane travel can cause a sinus headache. Signs and symptoms include:

- Pain in your forehead, cheekbones, and nose. The pain is worse in the morning.

- Increased pain when you bend over or touch your face.

- Stuffy nose.

Other Causes of Headaches

- Analgesic rebound from regular or repeated use of over-the-counter or prescribed pain relievers.

- Eating or drinking something very cold, such as ice cream. {*Note:* To prevent ice cream headaches, warm the ice cream for a few seconds in the front of your mouth.}

- Low blood sugar. Hunger.

- Cigarette smoke or exposure to chemicals and/or pollution.

- Uncorrected vision problems, such as nearsightedness.

- Caffeine withdrawal.

- Temporomandibular Joint (TMJ) Syndrome.

A headache can be a symptom of other health conditions. Examples are allergies, depression (see page 20), infections, and dental problems.

Treatment

Self-care can treat headaches caused by tension, fatigue, and/or stress. Certain over-the-counter medicines and prescribed medicines can treat migraine headaches.

Biofeedback has helped many people who have suffered from headaches.

Headaches that are symptoms of health conditions are relieved when the condition is treated with success.

Questions to Ask

Is the headache associated with any of the following?
- A head injury.
- A blow to the head that causes severe pain, enlarged pupils, vomiting, confusion, or lethargy.
- Loss of consciousness.

YES Get Immediate Care

NO

Has the headache come on suddenly and does it hurt much more than any headache you have ever had?

YES Get Immediate Care

NO

Does a severe, persistent headache occur with any of the following **signs and symptoms of meningitis**?
- Stiff neck (can't bend the head forward to touch the chin to the chest).
- Red or purple rash that doesn't fade when pressure is applied to the skin.
- Seizure.
- Lethargy.

YES Get Immediate Care

NO

Has the headache been occurring for more than 2 to 3 days and does it keep increasing in frequency and intensity?

YES See Provider

NO

Flowchart continued in next column

Do you have **signs and symptoms of a migraine headache** listed on pages 35 and 36?

YES See Provider

NO

Is the headache not relieved by over-the-counter pain relievers and does it occur with any **signs and symptoms of a sinus infection** listed on page 17?

YES See Provider

NO

Has the headache occurred at the same time of day, week, or month, such as with a menstrual period and is it not relieved by over-the-counter pain relievers?

YES See Provider

NO

Do you have to take a pain reliever more than 3 times a week for at least 3 weeks for headaches?

YES Call Provider

NO

Have you noticed the headache only after taking newly prescribed or over-the-counter medicines?

YES Call Provider

NO

 Use Self-Care

See Self-Care on next page

Common Health Problems

Headaches, *Continued*

Self-Care

- Take an over-the-counter medicine for pain as directed on the label. (See "**Pain Relievers**" in "**Over-the-Counter Medication Safety**" on page 75.)

- Rest in a quiet, dark room with your eyes closed.

- Massage the back of your neck with your thumbs. Work from the ears toward the center of the back of your head. Also, rub gently along the sides of your eyes. Gently rub your shoulders, neck, and jaw. Get a massage.

- Take a warm bath or shower.

- Place a cold or warm washcloth or OTC hot or cold pack over the area that aches.

- Relax. Picture a calm scene in your head. Meditate or breathe deeply.

- Avoid things that seem to bring on headaches.

- Try using a different pillow and/or sleep position.

- If you grind your teeth, tell your dentist or doctor.

- For a hangover: After drinking alcohol, take an over-the-counter pain reliever. Eat solid foods. Rest or sleep. Have 2 or more glasses of water before you go to sleep. Drink 2 or more glasses of water when you wake up.

For Information, Contact:

National Headache Foundation
800.843.2256
www.headaches.org

Skin Injuries

"I burned my hand pretty bad this year cooking, I dropped the potholder right before grabbing the oven rack! I put cold water and ice on it. It kept blistering and burning anyway. I ended up going to the Health Center. The nurse gave me something to put on the burn. It helped a lot."

Aimee S., Franklin Pierce College

Skin injuries can be as minor as a simple scrape or as major as a 3rd degree burn. The quicker you treat an injury, the faster the healing occurs.

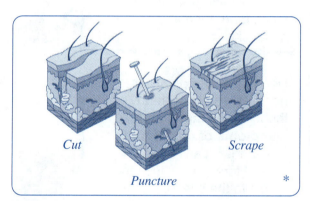

Cut   *Scrape*

Puncture   *

Signs, Symptoms & Causes

The signs, symptoms, and causes of skin injuries vary depending on the type of injury.

- **Cuts** – Cuts slice the skin open. This causes bleeding and pain. Cuts need to be cleaned, closed, and covered with a bandage so they don't get infected. Stitches may be needed for cuts that are deep, are longer than an inch, or are in an area of the body that bends, such as the elbow or knee. When appropriate, a topical tissue adhesive may be used instead of stitches to "super glue" the area.

Skin Injuries, *Continued*

- **Scrapes** – Scrapes are less serious than cuts, but hurt more because more sensitive nerve endings are involved.

- **Punctures** – Punctures are stab wounds. They can be shallow ones, such as from a splinter or deep ones, such as from stepping on a nail. Puncture wounds hurt and bleed.

- **Bruises** – Bruises are caused by broken blood vessels that bleed into the tissue under the skin. Common causes are falls or being hit by some force. A bruise causes black and blue or red skin. As it heals, the skin turns yellowish-green. Pain or tenderness and possible swelling also occur.

- **Burns** – Burns can be caused from dry heat (fire), moist heat (steam, hot liquids), electricity, chemicals, and the sun (sunburn).

  - With a 1st degree burn, your skin will be red, swollen, painful, and sensitive to touch. This usually heals in 1 to 2 days.

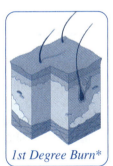

*1st Degree Burn**

  - With a 2nd degree burn, the outer and lower skin layers are affected. Your skin will be painful, swollen, red, blistered, and/or be weepy/watery.

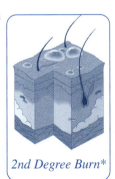

*2nd Degree Burn**

- With a 3rd degree burn, your skin will be black and white and charred. You will have less pain because the nerves have been destroyed.

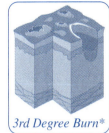

*3rd Degree Burn**

- **Animal and Human Bites** – Common symptoms are pain and bleeding. Wounds from animal and human bites can easily get infected. Rabies can result if the bite was from a warm-blooded animal who was infected with the rabies virus.

Treatment

Treatment varies depending on the cause and how severe the injury is. Simple wounds can be treated with self-care. An antibiotic is prescribed for an infection.

Questions to Ask

Do the following **signs of shock** occur with an injury?
- Pale or blue-colored lips, skin, and/or fingernails.
- Cool and moist skin.
- Weak, but fast pulse.
- Rapid, shallow breathing.
- Weakness, trembling, restlessness, confusion.
- Difficulty standing or inability to stand due to dizziness.
- Loss of consciousness.

YES Get Immediate Care

NO

Does an animal bite cause severe bleeding or severely mangled skin or has a human bite punctured the skin?

YES Get Immediate Care

NO

Flowchart continued on next page

Skin Injuries, *Continued*

Flowchart continued

Are any of these problems present?

- Severe bleeding or blood spurts from the wound. (Apply direct pressure on the wound site while seeking care.)
- Bleeding continues after pressure has been applied for more than 10 minutes (or after 20 minutes to what seems to be a minor cut).
- A deep cut or puncture appears to go down to the muscle or bone and/or is located on the scalp or face.
- A cut is longer than an inch and is located on an area of the body that bends, such as the elbow, knee, or finger.
- The skin on the edges of the cut hangs open.
- A burn (3rd degree) results in charred black and white skin, little or no pain, and exposure of tissue under the skin.
- A burn (2nd degree) causes painful, swollen, and red skin with blisters that cover more than 10 square inches of skin area or is on the face, hands, feet, genitals, or any joint.

YES 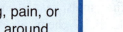 Get Immediate Care

NO

Flowchart continued in next column

Was the bite from a pet that has not been immunized against rabies or from an animal known to carry rabies in your area? (Check with your local health department, hospital, or emergency department if you are not sure.)

YES Get Immediate Care

NO

A day or two after the skin injury, do one or more of these **signs of an infection** occur?

- Fever and a general ill feeling.
- Redness or red streaks that extend from the wound site.
- Increased swelling, pain, or tenderness at and around the wound site.

YES See Provider

NO

Was the cut or puncture from dirty or contaminated objects, such as rusty nails or objects in the soil or did a puncture go through a shoe, especially a rubber-soled one? {*Note:* You will need a tetanus shot if you have not had one within 10 years.}

YES See Provider

NO

Flowchart continued on next page

Skin Injuries, *Continued*

Flowchart continued

With a skin injury, are any of the following conditions present?
- With a second-degree burn, more than the outer skin layer has been affected; more than 3 inches in diameter of the skin has been burned; or blisters have formed.
- The burn does not improve in 48 hours.
- Bruises appear often and easily; take longer than 2 weeks to heal; or ovor a year's time, more than 3 bruises appear for no apparent reason.
- Vision problems occur with a bruise near the eye.

YES →
See Provider

NO ↓

Use Self-Care

Self-Care

For Human Bites Before Immediate Care

- Wash the wound area with soap and water for at least 5 minutes, but don't scrub hard.

- Rinse the wound area with running water or with an antiseptic solution, such as Betadine.

- Cover the wound area with sterile gauze, taping only the ends in place.

{*Note:* All human bites need immediate care.}

For Minor Cuts and Scrapes

- Clean in and around the wound thoroughly with soap and water.

- Press on the cut to stop the bleeding for up to 10 minutes. Use sterile, wet gauze or a clean cloth. Dry gauze can stick to the wound. Don't use a bandage to apply pressure.

- If still bleeding, press on the cut again. Get medical help if it still bleeds after applying pressure for 10 more minutes. Lift the part of the body with the cut higher than the heart, if practical.

- After the bleeding has stopped, and when it is clean and dry, apply a first-aid cream.

- Put one or more bandages on the cut. The edges of the cut skin should touch, but not overlap. Use a butterfly bandage if you have one.

- Keep a scrape clean and dry. Dress it with gauze and first-aid tape. Change the bandage every 24 hours.

For Punctures that Cause Minor Bleeding

- Let the wound bleed to cleanse itself.

- Remove the object that caused the puncture. Use clean, sterile tweezers. To sterilize them, hold a lit match or flame to the ends of the tweezers. Let them cool and wipe the ends with sterile gauze. {*Note:* Don't pull anything out of a puncture wound if blood gushes from it or it has been bleeding badly. Get emergency care!}

- Two to 4 times a day, clean the wound area with warm, soapy water. Dry it well and apply an antibacterial cream. Do this for several days.

Common Health Problems

Skin Injuries, *Continued*

For Bruises

- Apply a cold pack to the bruised area as soon as possible (within 15 minutes of the injury). Keep the cold pack on for 10 minutes at a time. Apply pressure to the cold pack. Take it off for 30 to 60 minutes. Repeat several times for 2 days.

- Rest the bruised area and raise it above the level of the heart, if practical.

- Two days after the injury, use warm compresses for 20 minutes at a time.

- Do not bandage a bruise.

- Try to avoid hitting the bruised area again.

For First-Degree Burns and Second-Degree Burns (that are less than 3" in diameter):

- Use cold water or cloths soaked in cold water on burned areas for 15 minutes or until the pain subsides. Do not use ice at all; it could cause frostbite.

- Cover the area loosely with a clean dry cloth, such as sterile gauze. Hold it in place by taping only the edges of the gauze. Change the dressing the next day and every 2 days after that.

- Don't use ointments. You can apply aloe vera over closed skin 3 to 4 times a day .

- Don't break blisters. If they break on their own, apply an antibacterial spray or ointment. Or, use the treatment prescribed by your doctor. Keep the area loosely covered with a sterile dressing.

- For a severe burn less than 3 inches by 2 inches, use Second Skin Moisture Pads, etc.

- Prop the burned area higher than the rest of the body, if you can.

For Dog and Cat Bites

- To remove any saliva and other debris, wash the bite area right away with soap and warm water for 5 minutes. If the bite is deep, flush the wound with water for 10 minutes. Dry the wound with a clean towel. Then get immediate care.

- If the wound is swollen, apply ice wrapped in a towel for 10 minutes.

- A tetanus shot is needed if tetanus immunizations are not up-to-date.

- If the bite hurts, take an over-the-counter medicine for pain.

- Report the incident to the animal control department.

- If you know the pet's owner, find out the date of the pet's last rabies vaccination. If its immunizations are not current, arrange with the animal control department for the pet to be observed for the next 10 days to be sure it does not develop rabies.

- Observe the wound for a few days, checking it for signs of infection.

{*Note:* For all bites, cuts, scrapes, punctures, and burns, be sure your tetanus shot is up-to-date. Call your health care provider or your school's health service to check.}

For Information, Contact:

MedlinePlus® Health Information
www.medlineplus.gov
Search for "First Aid / Emergencies."

Sore Throats

"Cheering at the game was great, but my voice was hoarse and my throat was sore the next couple of days."

Chris B., Duke University

Sore throats are common complaints of college students. The soreness can range from a mere scratch to severe pain.

Signs & Symptoms

- Dry, irritated throat.
- Soreness or pain in the throat, especially when you talk or swallow.
- Swollen neck glands.
- The back of the throat and/or the tonsils look bright red or have pus deposits or white spots.
- Enlarged tonsils that feel tender (tonsillitis).

You may have other symptoms with the sore throat, too. These include fatigue, fever, postnasal drip, bad breath, headache, and/or earache.

Causes

- Viruses, such as with a cold or the flu or mononucleosis.
- A bacterial infection, such as strep throat.
- Shouting for long periods of time, such as from cheering at a sporting event.
- Tobacco or marijuana smoke.
- Dry air. Allergies. Cough. Postnasal drip.
- Self-induced vomiting.
- An infection from oral sex with an infected partner.

A rapid strep test can tell if you have strep bacteria. (Find out if your school offers this without having to see your health care provider).

Treatment

Self-care treats most sore throats. If strep is found, an antibiotic will be prescribed. Take all of the antibiotic to help prevent other conditions, such as rheumatic fever. Sore throats caused by viruses **do not** need an antibiotic.

Questions to Ask

With a sore throat, do you have severe shortness of breath or are you unable to swallow your own saliva?

YES → Get Immediate Care

NO ↓

With a sore throat, do you have any of these problems?
- Fever, chills, nausea, headache, and swollen, enlarged neck glands.
- Ear pain that persists.
- A bad smell from the throat, nose, or ears.
- Skin rash.
- Dark urine.

YES → See Provider

NO ↓

Do your tonsils or does the back of your throat look bright red or have pus deposits?

YES → See Provider

NO ↓

Flowchart continued on next page

 To Learn More, See Back Cover

Common Health Problems

Common Health Problems

Sore Throats, *Continued*

Flowchart continued

Does your roommate or others you live with have strep throat or do you get strep throat or tonsillitis often? **YES** → See Provider

NO

Has even a mild sore throat lasted more than 3 weeks? **YES** → Call Provider

NO

Use Self-Care

Self-Care

To Prevent Getting a Sore Throat

■ Do not get in close contact with anyone you know who has a sore throat.

■ Wash your hands often to minimize picking up germs from others. Also, don't share drinking glasses and silverware.

To Treat a Sore Throat

■ Gargle every 2 to 3 hours with a solution of ¼ teaspoon of salt mixed in 1 cup of warm water.

■ Drink plenty of warm beverages, such as tea with lemon (with or without honey) and soup.

■ For strep throat, have cold foods and liquids.

■ Use a cool-mist vaporizer in your room. If you get a sore throat often, consider putting a portable air purifier in your room.

■ Don't smoke. Avoid secondhand smoke and air pollution.

■ Avoid eating spicy foods.

■ Suck on a piece of hard candy, cough drop, or medicated lozenge every 2 to 4 hours.

■ Take an over-the-counter medicine for the pain and/or fever. (See "**Pain Relievers**" in "**Over-the-Counter Medication Safety**" on page 75.)

■ If prescribed an antibiotic, take all of it.

Sprains, Strains & Sports Injuries

"We were playing football on a Saturday afternoon when one guy dislocated a shoulder. You could tell because it was 3 inches lower than the other shoulder. We iced it and took him to the health service."

Daniel P., University of the Pacific

Signs, Symptoms & Causes

Sprains

A sprain happens when you overstretch or tear a ligament (fibrous tissue that connects bones). A joint is affected, but there is no dislocation or fracture.

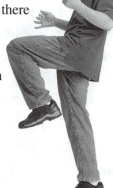

Symptoms are rapid pain, swelling, bruising, and a warm feeling at the injured site.

Sprains usually occur from an accident, injury, or fall.

Sprains, Strains & Sports Injuries, *Continued*

Strains

A strain is an injury to the muscles or tendons (tissues that connect muscles to bones). Symptoms are pain, tenderness, swelling, and bruising. A strain occurs when you overstretch or overexert a muscle or tendon (not a ligament). This is usually caused by overuse and injuries, such as sports injuries.

Sports Injuries

- Achilles tendon pain is caused by a stretch or tear or irritation to the tendon that connects the calf muscles to the back of the heel.

- Blisters are due to friction, such as from poor fitting shoes or socks.

- Muscle soreness occurs when you have worked out too hard and too long.

- Shinsplints are mild to severe aches in front of the lower leg.

- Stress fractures are microfractures which usually involve the bones of the feet or legs. They are usually caused by a sudden increase in the amount of weight bearing exercise being done.

Sports injury symptoms vary depending on the injury. They include pain, tenderness, swelling, and bruising. Bones may be broken or dislocated.

Treatment

Treatment depends on the injury and the extent of damage. Self-care may suffice for mild injuries.

Sports injuries and sprains may need medical treatment. Some sprains require a cast. Others may need surgery if the tissue affected is torn.

Broken bones (other than broken toes) need immediate medical care.

Questions to Ask

Do you suspect a head, neck, or spinal injury by any of these symptoms?
- The person has lost consciousness.
- Inability to move the head, neck, or back.
- Inability to open and close the fingers or move the toes or any part of the arms or legs.
- Feelings of numbness in the legs, arms, shoulders, or any other part of the body.
- It looks like the head, neck, or back is in an odd position.
- Immediate neck pain.
  {**Note:** If any of the above problems exist, tell the person to lie still and not move his or her head, neck, back, etc. Place rolled towels, articles of clothing, etc. on both sides of the neck and/or body. Tie and wrap them in place, but don't interfere with the person's breathing. If necessary, use both of your hands, one on each side of the person's head, to keep the head from moving. Call 9-1-1!}

YES Get Immediate Care

NO

Flowchart continued on next page

 To Learn More, See Back Cover

Common Health Problems

Sprains, Strains & Sports Injuries, *Continued*

Flowchart continued

Did a strain or sprain occur with great force from a vehicle accident or a fall from a high place?

YES → **Get Immediate Care**

NO

Are any of these signs present?
- A bone sticks out or bones in the injured part make a grating sound.
- An injured body part looks bent, shortened, or misshaped.
- You can't move the injured body part or put weight on it.
- The injured area is blue, pale, or feels cool, but the same limb on the other side of the body does not.

YES → **Get Immediate Care**

NO

Are any of these signs present?
- You can't bend or straighten an injured limb.
- Bad pain and swelling occur or the pain gets worse.
- Pain is felt when you press along the bone near the injury.

YES → **See Provider**

{Note: If you are in a sports program and you have an injury, contact your trainer.}

NO

Does the sprain or strain not improve after using self-care measures for 2 days?

YES → **Call Provider**

NO

 Use Self-Care

Self-Care

To Prevent Serious Injuries (especially during contact sports)

- Wear the right protective gear and clothing for the sport. Items to wear include a helmet, shoulder, knee, and wrist pads, a mouth guard, etc.

- Train in the sport so you learn how to avoid injury. "Weekend athletes" are prone to injury.

- Follow the rules that apply to the sport.

General Prevention

- Ease into any exercise program. Increase activity gradually.

- Do warm-up stretching exercises before the activity. Stretch and hold for at least 30 seconds. Don't bounce.

- Wear proper-fitting shoes that provide shock absorption and stability.

- Avoid running on hard surfaces like asphalt and concrete. Run on flat surfaces instead of uphill. Running uphill aggravates the stress put on the Achilles tendon.

- Use the softest surface available when you exercise.

- Wear shoes and socks that fit well. The widest area of your foot should match the widest area of the shoe. You should also be able to wiggle your toes with the shoe on, in both a sitting and standing position. The inner seams of the shoe should not rub against areas of your feet.

- Avoid locking your knees. When jumping, land with your knees bent.

- Don't overdo it. Stop if you feel pain.

Sprains, Strains & Sports Injuries, *Continued*

■ Cool down after exercise. Do the activity at a slower pace for 5 minutes.

To Treat a Sprain, Strain, or Sports Injury

■ If the injury does not appear serious, stop what you are doing and use **R.I.C.E.**:

Rest the injured area for 24 to 48 hours.

Ice the injured area as soon as possible and keep doing so for 10 minutes every 2 hours for the next 48 hours. Use an ice pack, ice in a heavy plastic bag with a little water, a bag of frozen vegetables, etc.

Compress the area. Wrap with an elastic bandage. Numbness, tingling, or increased pain means the bandage is too tight. Remove the bandage every 3 to 4 hours and leave it off for 15 to 20 minutes each time.

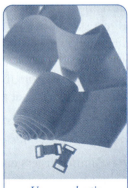

Use an elastic bandage to compress the injured area.

Elevate the injured area above heart level, if possible.

■ Take an over-the-counter medicine for pain, if necessary. (See "**Pain Relievers**" in "**Over-the-Counter Medication Safety**" on page 75).

{*Note:* Many sports medicine providers do not recommend aspirin-like medication at first because it can aggravate bleeding and bruising.}

■ If you sprained a finger or hand, remove rings. (If you don't and your fingers swell up, the rings may have to be cut off.)

■ Try liniments and balms. These provide a cooling or warming sensation. These ointments only mask the pain of sore muscles, though. They do not promote healing.

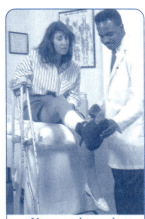

Use crutches only when it is too painful to bear weight.

■ Once the injured area begins to heal, do **M.S.A.** techniques:

Movement. Work to establish a full range of motion as soon as possible after an injury. This will help maintain flexibility during healing and prevent scar tissue formed by the injury from limiting future performance.

Strength. Gradually strengthen the injured area once the inflammation is controlled and a range of motion is back.

Alternative Activities. Do regular exercise using activities that do not strain the injured part. Start this a few days after the injury, even though the injured part is still healing.

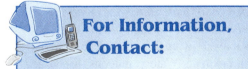

For Information, Contact:

MedlinePlus® Health Information
www.medlineplus.gov
Search for "First Aid/Emergencies."

Common Health Problems

STIs/HIV

Sexually transmitted infections (STIs) are ones that pass from one person to another through sexual contact (e.g., vaginal, anal, and oral sex, and genital-to-genital contact). STIs are also called sexually transmitted diseases (STDs).

Seventy-five percent of STIs are acquired in persons who range in age from 15 to 24 years old.

Common STIs in the U.S. are: Chlamydia; genital herpes; gonorrhea; hepatitis B; HIV/AIDS; human papillomavirus (HPV) – the cause of genital warts; and trichomoniasis. The most common ones among college students are chlamydia and HPV.

Syphilis, another STI, is not as common as it used to be, but still exists. For information on this STI, access www.cdc.gov.

More than one STI can be present at the same time. Some can be present without symptoms. If you are sexually active or have ever had sex without adequate "barrier" protection (e.g. latex or polyurethane condom), you could have an STI and not even know it.

Signs, Symptoms & Causes

Chlamydia

Chlamydia is caused by different strains of the bacterium *chlamydia trachomatis*.

About 25 percent of males have few or no symptoms, but can still transmit the disease. Symptoms may show up 2 to 4 weeks after infection and include: Watery, mucous discharge from the penis; burning or discomfort when urinating; and pain in the scrotum.

Seventy-five percent of females have few or no symptoms, but can still transmit the disease.

When present, symptoms show up 2 to 4 weeks after infection and include: Slight yellowish-green vaginal discharge; vaginal irritation or pain or burning feeling when urinating; abdominal pain; and abnormal vaginal bleeding. In females, chlamydia can cause pelvic inflammatory disease (PID), which can cause infertility. (See **"Pelvic Inflammatory Disease" (PID)** on page 61.)

Genital Herpes

The Herpes simplex virus (HSV-1 or HSV-2) causes genital herpes. HSV-1 often affects the oral area, showing up as cold sores, but can affect the genital area, too. HSV-2 usually affects the genital area, upper thighs, and area near the anus, but can also affect the oral area. The virus is spread by direct skin-to-skin contact from the site of infection to the contact site, but can also be spread when no symptoms are noticed. Oral sex can spread herpes from the mouth to the genital area and from the genital area to the mouth.

Signs and symptoms (which may appear as early as 2 to 20 days after contact) include:

- Painful blisters and/or sores on the genital area, anus, and thighs and/or buttocks.

- Itching, irritation, and tingling in the genital area 1 to 2 days before the blisters appear.

- After a few days, the blisters break open and leave painful, shallow ulcers, which can last from 5 days to 3 weeks.

With outbreaks, especially the first one, there may be flu-like symptoms (swollen glands, fever, body aches). Outbreaks that follow are usually milder and shorter. Once infected, the virus lives in nerve cells and new outbreaks can occur even without contact. Stress, fatigue, illnesses, and sunburn may trigger outbreaks.

STIs/HIV, *Continued*

Using a latex or polyurethane barrier (condom, dental dam, etc.) when you have sex or skin-to-skin contact may help prevent transmission, but this is not guaranteed.

The sores may be located on skin areas not covered by the latex or polyurethane barrier. The virus can also be transmitted when sores are not present. This is known as "viral shedding."

Gonorrhea

Gonorrhea is also called "the clap," "dose," or "drip." It is caused by a specific bacterial infection. If not treated, it can spread to joints, tendons, or the heart. In females, it can cause pelvic inflammatory disease (PID), which is directly linked to infertility in females. (See **"Pelvic Inflammatory Disease (PID)"** on page 61.)

Sixty to 80% of females have no symptoms. If symptoms are present, they appear 2 to 10 days after infection and include: Mild vaginal itching and burning; thick, yellow-green vaginal discharge; burning when urinating; and severe pain in lower abdomen.

In males, signs and symptoms include: Pain at the tip of the penis; pain and burning during urination; and a thick, yellow, cloudy, penile discharge that gradually increases.

Hepatitis B

Hepatitis B is a virus that causes liver inflammation. The virus can be spread from contact with blood or bodily fluids from an infected person. Examples are having sex and/or sharing drug needles with an infected person and exposure to infected blood through cuts, open sores, and unsterilized instruments used for body piercing.

Sharing razors with an infected person and exposure to an infected person's saliva may transmit the virus. Hepatitis B is not spread through food or water or by casual contact.

Three doses of Hepatitis B vaccine can prevent getting this virus. Consult your health care provider if you have not yet received this vaccine.

Some persons have no symptoms. When symptoms first occur, they are flu-like (fatigue, fever, appetite loss, nausea and vomiting, and joint pain).

Later, symptoms include jaundice, dark urine, and pale, clay-colored stools.

HIV/AIDS

HIV stands for human immunodeficiency virus. AIDS, acquired immune deficiency syndrome, is caused by HIV. HIV destroys the body's immune system leaving a person unable to fight off diseases. The virus also attacks the central nervous system causing mental and neurological problems.

HIV is spread when body fluids, such as semen and blood, pass from an infected person to another person. Usually, the virus is spread by sexual contact or by sharing drug needles. It can also be passed from an infected female to her baby during childbirth or breast-feeding.

You cannot get HIV from donating blood, touching, hugging, or social (dry) kissing a person with HIV. You cannot get HIV from a cough, a sneeze, tears, sweat, or from

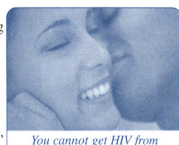

You cannot get HIV from hugging a person with HIV.

using a hot tub, telephone, or restroom.

STIs/HIV, *Continued*

Symptoms of HIV before the Onset of AIDS

- Swollen glands.
- Fatigue. Weight loss.
- Fever and sweating. These occur often.
- Skin rashes that persist. Flaky skin.
- Infections. These include herpes, shingles, and yeast infections.
- Short-term memory loss.
- Getting sick often.

When HIV invades the brain, impaired speech, trembling, and seizures can occur.

AIDS is the most advanced stage of HIV. With AIDS, a low level of cells in the blood called T4 cells occurs. Persons with AIDS get many illnesses. These include skin infections, tuberculosis, pneumonia, and cancer.

Human Papillomavirus (HPV) – Genital Warts

About 25 types of HPV can infect the genital area. Only a few types cause genital warts. Other types increase the risk for cervical cancer.

Often, there are no visible signs or symptoms. Genital warts are often skin-colored, do not hurt, and may be located inside the vagina or the head of the penis, or in the anus. This makes them hard to see. To find out if you have genital warts, a health care provider can put a solution of acetic acid (vinegar) on the genitals.

HPV is spread by direct skin-to-skin contact during vaginal, anal, or (rarely) oral sex with an infected partner. You don't get genital warts from touching warts on other parts of the body, such as the feet or hands.

Genital warts can appear several weeks after being infected or may not show up for months or even years. This makes it hard to know when the virus was acquired and which partner was the carrier.

Three doses of HPV vaccine can prevent the most common types of HPV that are associated with cervical cancer in females and genital warts in females and males. (See **Immunizations** on page 81).

You can also lower the risk for getting HPV by using latex or polyurethane condoms, which are more likely to cover potentially affected areas of the body. (A diaphragm will not prevent transmission.)

Trichomoniasis

Trichomoniasis is caused by a protozoan, not by bacteria or a virus.

In females, the protozoan can be present in the vagina for years without causing symptoms. If they do occur, typical symptoms include:

- Vaginal itching and burning.
- A yellow-green or gray vaginal discharge with an odor.
- Burning or pain when urinating.
- Painful sexual intercourse.

In males, symptoms are not usually present. Males may infect their sexual partners and not know it. When present, symptoms include:

- Discomfort when urinating.
- Pain during intercourse.
- Irritation and itching of the penis.

STIs/HIV, *Continued*

Treatment

Call your health care provider, your school's Health Service, or the National STD Hotline (800.227.8922) to find out how to get tested for STIs.

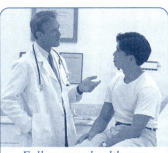

Follow your health care provider's advice.

Testing may be free at your college's Health Service. Treatment depends on proper diagnosis.

For Chlamydia

- Oral antibiotics for the infected person and his or her partner(s).

- Avoiding sex until treatment is completed in the infected person and his or her partner(s).

For Genital Herpes

- There is no cure. Symptoms occur, though, only during flare-ups.

- Oral antiviral medicines (e.g. acyclovir, valacyclovir) can help prevent outbreaks and shorten how long the outbreaks last.

- Self-Care measures listed on page 52.

For Gonorrhea

- Antibiotics.

- Pain relievers.

- Treating sexual partner(s) to avoid re-infection.

- Follow-up test to find out if the treatment was effective.

For Hepatitis B

- Self-Care measures on pages 52 and 53.

- Medication may be prescribed for chronic cases.

While most people with this type recover, up to 10% can become chronic. (The person can spread the infection even though he or she has no symptoms.) This type can lead to cirrhosis of the liver and liver failure in some persons.

For HIV/AIDS

- Medications. These are often used in multidrug combinations.

- Treating infections, such as pneumonia.

For HPV (Genital Warts)

- The warts can be treated with topical creams or a gel prescribed by a doctor. You apply these yourself.

- The warts can be removed medically by cryosurgery (freezing them); an acidic chemical that burns them; or laser surgery.

- Females who have had HPV should get Pap tests as often as advised by their health care providers to screen for signs of cervical cancer. These females should not smoke.

For Trichomoniasis

- The oral medication metronidazole (Flagyl). {*Note*: Don't drink alcohol for 24 hours before, during, and 24 hours after taking metronidazole. The combination causes vomiting, dizziness, and headaches.}

- Treating sexual partners to prevent spreading the infection and getting it again.

 To Learn More, See Back Cover

STIs/HIV, *Continued*

Questions to Ask

Do you test positive for HIV or do you have signs and symptoms of any STI listed in this topic? **YES** See Provider

NO

Do you already have a diagnosis of genital herpes and do you have severe pain and blistering and/or are you having outbreaks often? **YES** See Provider

NO

Are you symptom-free, but worried that you got an STI from someone you suspect may have one? **YES** See Provider

NO

Do you want to rule out an STI because you have had many sex partners and you are considering a new sexual relationship or planning to get married or pregnant? **YES** See Provider

NO

Do sores appear in the genital area only after taking a recently prescribed medicine? **YES** See Provider

NO

Use Self-Care

Self-Care continued in next column

Self-Care

Sexually transmitted infections need medical care. Along with medical care, do the following:

For Genital Herpes

- If prescribed an oral antiviral medicine, take it as directed.

- Bathe the affected area twice a day with mild soap and water. Pat dry with a towel or use a hair dryer set on warm. Using a colloidal oatmeal soap or bath may be soothing.

- Use a sitz bath to soak the affected area. You can buy a sitz bath basin from a medical supply or drug store.

- Apply ice packs on the affected genital area for 5 to 10 minutes to relieve itching and swelling.

- Wear loose fitting pants or skirts. Don't wear pantyhose. Wear cotton (not nylon) underwear.

- If pain is made worse when you urinate, squirt tepid water near the urinary opening while you pass urine or urinate while using a sitz bath.

- Take a mild pain reliever, as directed.

- Ask your doctor about using a local anesthetic ointment, such as lidocaine, during the most painful part of an outbreak.

- Wash your hands if you touch the blisters or sores. To avoid spreading the virus to your eyes, don't touch your eyes during an outbreak.

- To help avoid spreading the virus to others, use latex barriers during sex and skin-to-skin contact.

For Hepatitis B

- Rest. Drink at least 8 glasses of fluids a day.

- Avoid alcohol and any drugs or medicines that affect the liver, such as acetaminophen.

STIs/HIV, *Continued*

■ Follow a healthy diet. Take vitamin and mineral supplements as advised by your health care provider.

■ Use latex condoms during sexual intercourse to help avoid spreading the virus.

For HIV/AIDS

Medical care, not self-care alone, is needed to treat HIV/AIDS. Self-care measures include:

■ Taking steps to reduce the risk of getting infections and diseases:

• Get adequate rest and proper nutrition. Take vitamin supplements, as advised by your doctor.

• Get emotional support. Join a support group. Also ask your family and friends for support.

For Information, Contact:

AIDSinfo
800.HIV.0440 (448.0440)
www.aidsinfo.nih.gov

American Sexual Health Association (ASHA)
ASHA's STI Resource Center Hotline
919.361.8488
www.ashastd.org

CDC National AIDS Hotline (NAH)
800.CDC.INFO (232.4636)
CDC National STD Hotline
800.CDC.INFO (232.4636)
www.cdc.gov/std

Stress

"A friend of mine had 9 papers to write in 2 days. We all watched her eat 25 peanut butter cups and go into a strange laughing fit we called "crack up!"

Nancy M., University of Colorado

College years can be great fun. They can also be filled with a lot of stress. You have to deal with a lot of changes. These include:

■ Separation from home and friends.

■ Adjusting to a new place to live, which can be small, noisy, cluttered, and lack privacy.

■ Academic overload and financial demands.

■ Competition, fear of failure, and making career choices.

Stress is the way you react to these and other changes. Stress can make you more productive. It can make you study harder to get good grades. High stress levels, though, can make you less productive.

Signs & Symptoms

■ Physical symptoms of stress include increased heart rate and blood pressure, rapid breathing, tense muscles, sleeping poorly, and changes in appetite.

■ Emotional reactions include irritability, anger, losing your temper, and lack of concentration.

Treatment

Prevention and self-care measures deal with most cases of stress. When these are not enough, counseling and/or medical care may be needed. Counseling services at your school may be free.

Common Health Problems

Stress, *Continued*

Questions to Ask

Are you so distressed that you have recurrent thoughts of suicide or death and/or do you have impulses or plans to commit violence? **YES** Get Immediate Care

NO

Are you abusing alcohol and/or drugs (illegal or prescription) to deal with stress? **YES** See Provider

NO

Do you have any of these problems often?
• Anxiety.
• Nervousness.
• Crying spells.
• Confusion about how to handle your problems. **YES** See Provider

NO

Do you withdraw from friends, relatives, and coworkers and/or blow up at them at the slightest annoyance? **YES** See Provider

NO

Are you unable to cope with a medical problem or does it cause so much stress that you neglect to get proper treatment for it? **YES** See Provider

NO

Flowchart continued in next column

Have you been a part of a traumatic event in the past (e.g. rape or assault) and now experience any of the following?
• Flashbacks (reliving the stressful event), painful memories, nightmares.
• Feeling easily startled and/or irritable.
• Feeling "emotionally numb" and detached from others and the outside world.
• Having a hard time falling asleep and/or staying asleep.
• Anxiety and/or depression. **YES** See Provider

NO

Use Self-Care

Self-Care

■ Listen to music that you find soothing while at a quiet, calm place. Meditate.

■ Get regular exercise.

■ Get as much sleep and rest as you can.

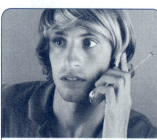

Talk about your troubles with a family member, a friend, etc., who will listen without judging.

■ Drink 8 to 10 glasses of water each day.

■ Reduce noise in your environment.

■ Eat healthy foods. Eat at regular times. Don't skip meals.

Stress, *Continued*

- Take a vitamin/mineral supplement that gives 100% of "Daily Values" for nutrients. Don't take ones marked "Stress Formula" on the label. High doses of some nutrients in these, such as vitamin B_6, can be harmful.

- Limit caffeine. It causes anxiety and increases the stress response. Avoid nicotine and other stimulants, such as No-Doz and diet pills.

- Balance work and play. Plan social and extracurricular activities in the time you have left after class, work, and sleep. Don't take on more activities than you can reasonably do in a given day or week. Set priorities.

- Take charge. Although you can't control other people's actions, you can control your response.

- Don't try to please everyone. You can't.

- Set up and maintain good study habits. Get prepared for tests and papers throughout the course of the class so you don't need to cram for them the night before they are due.

- Reward yourself with little things that make you feel good.

- Help others.

- Don't suppress having a good cry. Tears can help cleanse the body of substances that form under stress. Tears also release a natural pain-relieving substance from the brain.

- Do relaxation exercises daily. Good ones include visualization (imagining a soothing, restful scene), deep muscle relaxation (tensing and relaxing muscle fibers), meditation, and deep breathing.

- Count to 10 when you're so upset you want to scream. This gives you time to reflect on what's bothering you and helps to calm you down.

- Modify your environment to get rid of or manage your exposure to stress.

- Rehearse for stressful events. Imagine yourself feeling calm and confident in an anticipated stressful situation.

- View changes as positive challenges. Don't get down on yourself if you don't do well on a test. Plan to be better prepared next time. Ask your academic advisor or others for help.

- When a difficult problem is out of control, accept it until changes can be made.

- Escape for a little while. Watch a movie, etc.

- Laugh a lot. Keep a sense of humor.

- Take a warm shower or bath.

- Don't drink alcohol or take drugs to deal with stress. Have a warm cup of herbal tea.

For Information, Contact:

Your school's Student Affairs Office, Financial Aid Office, Career Development Office, etc.

Your school's Student Counseling Service, Mental Health Service, or Student Health Service

Stress Management and Emotional Wellness Links
www.howtostudy.com
www.goaskalice.columbia.edu

Suicidal Thoughts

"I've had feelings of just wanting to disappear. It's more than depression, like a complete giving up of life and all of its routine tasks."

Kim T., University of Wisconsin

For persons 15 to 24 years old, suicide is the third leading cause of death, behind unintentional injury and homicide. More teenagers and young adults die from suicide than from cancer, heart disease, AIDS, birth defects, stroke, pneumonia, influenza, and chronic lung disease *combined*. Young women attempt suicide 4 to 8 times more often than young men, but males are 4 times more likely than females to die from suicide.

Signs & Symptoms

A lot of people think about suicide or say things like, "I wish I was dead," at times of great stress. For most people, these thoughts are a way to express anger and other emotions. They may not, in and of themselves, be a sign of a problem. The signs and symptoms that follow need medical care.

- Writing a suicide note.
- Suicidal threats, gestures, or attempts.
- Thoughts of suicide that don't go away or that occur often.

(*Note:* In some suicides, no warning signs are shown or noticed.)

Causes

- Depression.
- Bipolar disorder.
- Schizophrenia.
- Grief. Loss of a loved one
- A side effect of some medicines. One is isotretinoin. This is presc for severe acne. Some antidepressant medicines can increase the risk for suicidal thoughts and behaviors, too. This is especially noted in children and adolescents. This risk may be higher within the first days to a month after starting the medicine. Persons who take antidepressants should be closely monitored.
- A family history of suicide or depression.
- Money and relationship problems.

Treatment

Suicidal threats and attempts are a person's way of letting others know that he or she needs help. They should never be taken lightly or taken only as a "bluff." Most people who threaten and/or attempt suicide more than once usually succeed if they are not stopped. Emergency care and hospitalization are necessary after an attempted suicide. Persons with suicidal thoughts should seek medical treatment.

Suicidal Thoughts, *Continued*

Questions to Ask

*{**Note:** In some suicides, no warning signs are shown or noticed.}*

At this time, are any of the following present?
- Suicide attempts or gestures, such as standing on the edge of a bridge, cutting the wrists, or driving recklessly on purpose.
- Plans are being made for suicide. Has the person purchased or gotten a weapon or pills that could be used for suicide?
- Repeated thoughts of suicide or death.

YES → **Get Immediate Care**

NO ↓

Has the person recently done any of the following?
- Given repeated statements that indicate suicidal thoughts, such as "I don't want to live anymore," or "The world would be better off without me."
- Given away things he or she values most and gotten legal matters in order.
- Suddenly felt better after being very depressed and stated something like, "Now I know what I have to do."

YES → **See Provider**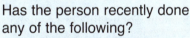

NO ↓

Flowchart continued in next column

With thoughts of suicide or death, are any of these conditions present?
- Depression or bipolar disorder.
- Schizophrenia.
- Any other mental health or medical condition.

YES → **See Provider**

NO ↓

Have thoughts of suicide occurred after taking, stopping, or changing the dose of a prescribed medicine (this includes certain antidepressants) or using drugs and/or alcohol?

YES → **See Provider**

NO ↓

Does the person thinking about suicide have **signs and symptoms of depression** (see page 20)?

YES → **See Provider**

NO ↓

Does the person thinking about suicide have other blood relatives who attempted or died from suicide?

YES → **See Provider**

NO ↓

Have suicidal thoughts come as a result of any of the following (or any other) upsets in life?
- A relationship breakup.
- The death of a loved one.
- A rejection or being ridiculed.

YES → **See Provider**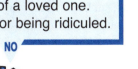

NO ↓

Use Self-Care

Self-Care continued on next page

Suicidal Thoughts, *Continued*

Self-Care

If You Are Having Thoughts of Suicide

- Let someone know. Talk to a trusted family member, friend, or teacher. If it is hard for you to talk directly to someone, write your thoughts down and let someone else read them.

- Call your school's Mental Health Service, your local Crisis Intervention Center or the National Suicide Prevention Lifeline at 800.273.8255. Follow up with a visit to your health care provider or your school's Mental Health Service.

How to Help a Friend Who May Be Suicidal

- Take him or her seriously. If your friend informs you of suicidal intentions, believe the threats.

- Keep firearms, drugs, etc. away from persons at risk.

- Take courses that teach problem solving, coping skills, and suicide awareness.

- If you think the person is serious about suicide, get help. Watch and protect him or her until you get help. Keep the person talking. Ask questions, such as, "Are you thinking about hurting or killing yourself?"

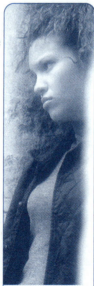

While getting help, do not leave a person alone who threatens suicide.

- Urge the person to call for help. If he or she is already under the care of a health care provider, have the person contact that provider first. If not, other places to contact are listed in the box below. Make the call yourself if the person can't or won't.

- Express concern. The person needs to know that someone cares. Most suicidal persons feel alone. Tell the person how much he or she means to you and others. Talk about reasons to stay alive. Don't judge. The person needs someone to listen, not to preach moral values.

- Tell the person that depression and suicidal tendencies can be treated. Urge him or her to get professional care. Offer help in seeking care.

For Information, Contact:

Your school's Student Counseling or Mental Health Service or Student Health Service

Your local Suicide Prevention Hotline or Crisis Intervention Center

American Foundation for Suicide Prevention 888.333.AFSP (2377) • www.afsp.org (This is not a crisis hotline.)

Metanoia Communications www.metanoia.org/suicide

National Suicide Prevention Lifeline 800.273.TALK (273.8255) www.suicidepreventionlifeline.org

Urinary Tract Infections (UTIs)

"I threw up twice during class and 3 times on the bus on the way back to my dorm. I thought I had the stomach flu. Then I felt really out of it. Luckily, my roommate was in pre-med. She got me to the University Medical Center's Emergency Room. I was dehydrated and I had a kidney infection."

Diana K., University of Michigan

Urinary tract infections are ones that occur in any organs that make up the urinary tract. The kidneys filter waste products from the blood and make urine. Ureters connect the kidney to the bladder, which holds urine until it is passed through the urethra.

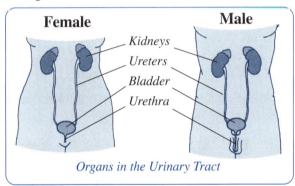

Female   **Male**

Kidneys
Ureters
Bladder
Urethra

Organs in the Urinary Tract

Signs & Symptoms

Bladder Infection

- Constant urge to urinate; urinating more often than usual; feeling like your bladder is still full after you pass urine.

- Burning or pain when you pass urine.

- Cloudy urine or blood in the urine.

Acute Kidney Infection

- Pain in one or both sides of your mid-back.

- Fever and shaking chills.

- Nausea and vomiting.

{*Note*: *Bladder infections are much more common than kidney infections*. You can also have a UTI without symptoms.}

Causes & Risk Factors

UTIs result when bacteria infect any part of the urinary tract. The bladder is the most common site.

The risk for getting a UTI is greater for:

- Sexually active females.

- Females who use a diaphragm.

- Males and females who have had UTIs in the past.

- Anyone with a condition that doesn't allow urine to pass freely. Kidney stones is an example.

Prevention

- Drink plenty of water and other fluids everyday. Cranberry juice may help prevent bladder infections.

- Empty your bladder as soon as you feel the urge.

- Drink a glass of water before you have sex. Go to the bathroom as soon as you can after sex.

- If you're prone to UTIs, don't take bubble baths.

- If you're female, wipe from front to back after using the toilet. This helps keep bacteria away from the opening of the urethra.

- If you use a diaphragm, clean it after each use. Have your health care provider check it periodically to make sure it still fits right.

Urinary Tract Infections (UTIs), *Continued*

Treatment

An antibiotic to treat the specific infection and pain relievers (if necessary) are the usual treatment. If you get UTIs often, your health care provider may order certain medical tests to diagnose the cause.

Questions to Ask

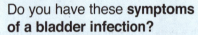

Do you have <u>all</u> of these **symptoms of a kidney infection?**
- Fever and shaking chills.
- Pain in one or both sides of your mid-back.
- Nausea and vomiting.

YES → Get Immediate Care

NO ↓

Do you have these **symptoms of a bladder infection?**
- Burning or stinging feeling when you pass urine.
- Passing urine a lot more often than usual, often in small amounts.
- Bloody, cloudy, or foul-smelling urine.
- Pain in your abdomen or over your bladder.
- Fever (sometimes).

YES → See Provider

NO ↓

Have you had more than 3 bladder infections within 6 months or more than 4 bladder infections in the same year?

YES → See Provider

NO ↓

Flowchart continued in next column

After taking prescribed medicine for a UTI, do symptoms not clear up over 3 days? Or, did the prescribed medicine give you side effects, such as a skin rash or a vaginal yeast infection (see page 61)?

YES → Call Provider

NO ↓

 Use Self-Care

Self-Care

- Drink at least 8 glasses of water and other liquids a day.

- Drink juice made from unsweetened cranberry juice concentrate. Take cranberry tablets. (Look for these at health food stores.)

- Avoid alcohol, spicy foods, and caffeine. These can irritate the bladder.

- Get plenty of rest.

- Take an over-the-counter medicine for pain. (see "**Pain Relievers**" in "**Over-the-Counter Medication Safety**" on page 75) or take the OTC medicine Uristat, which relieves pain and spasms that come with a bladder infection. {*Note:* Uristat helps with symptoms, but doesn't get rid of the infection. You should see your health care provider to diagnose and treat the problem.}

- Go to the bathroom as soon as you feel the urge. Empty your bladder completely.

- Don't have sexual intercourse until the infection is cleared up.

Vaginal Problems

"I just learned that yogurt could help to prevent yeast infections. Now when I take antibiotics, I eat a yogurt in the morning."

Kim P., University of Maryland

Vaginal problems include vaginal pain, discharge, abnormal bleeding, irritation, and/or infections. Infections may or may not be sexually transmitted. Common vaginal problems in college age females are listed below.

Signs, Symptoms & Causes

Bacterial Vaginosis

This is an infection from one or more types of bacteria. With this you may have:

- Mild vaginal irritation or burning.
- A thin, gray or milky white vaginal discharge with a fishy odor.

Pelvic Inflammatory Disease (PID)

This is an infection that goes up through the uterus to the fallopian tubes. Signs and symptoms are:

- Abdominal tenderness and/or bloating.
- Pain in the abdomen or back. The pain can be severe or it can occur midway in the menstrual cycle or during a pelvic exam.
- Pain during sex.
- Menstrual cramps can be very painful.
- The skin on your abdomen feels sensitive.
- Vaginal discharge with abnormal color or odor.
- Change in menstrual flow.
- Fever. Nausea.

Vaginal Yeast Infection

This is caused by an overgrowth of the fungus *Candida*. This is normally present in harmless amounts in the vagina, digestive tract, and mouth. Taking some brands of birth control pills and/or an antibiotic may trigger this overgrowth.

Symptoms of a vaginal yeast infection are:

- Thick, white vaginal discharge that looks like cottage cheese and may smell like yeast.
- Itching, irritation, and redness around the vagina.
- Burning and/or pain when passing urine or with sex.

Vaginitis From Contact Dermatitis

This is a reaction to products that irritate the vaginal area, such as harsh detergents, scented items, douches, latex condoms, and tight-fitting clothing. With this, itching and redness occur in the outer genital area without other symptoms.

Sexually Transmitted Infections

These include genital herpes, genital warts, gonorrhea, and trichomoniasis. (For signs and symptoms of these **Sexually Transmitted Infections**, see pages 48 to 50.)

Treatment

Treatment for the vaginal problem depends on the cause. Bacterial infections and PID are treated with antibiotics. Fungal infections are treated with antifungal medicines.

Common Health Problems

Vaginal Problems, *Continued*

Questions to Ask

Has a recent sexual assault or major injury to the abdomen, pelvis, or vagina occurred? **YES** Get Immediate Care

NO

Do you have vaginal pain that spreads upward to the pelvis and are you unable to walk due to the pain? **YES** Get Immediate Care

NO

Does vaginal irritation and/or pain occur with all of the **symptoms of a kidney infection** listed on page 60? **YES** Get Immediate Care

NO

Do you have very heavy vaginal bleeding (you saturate more than 1 full size pad or super absorbent tampon in an hour's time) with any of the following problems?

- Feeling dizzy, faint, or lightheaded when you sit up.
- Pale and moist skin.
- Extreme shortness of breath or a very hard time breathing.
- Severe abdominal pain.

YES 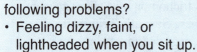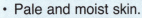 Get Immediate Care

NO

Flowchart continued in next column

Do you have any of the following?

- **Signs and symptoms of Pelvic Inflammatory Disease (PID)** listed on page 61.
- **Signs and symptoms of bacterial vaginosis** listed on page 61.
- **Signs and symptoms of a sexually transmitted infection** listed on pages 48 to 50.

YES See Provider

NO

Do any of the following apply?

- You have had 3 or more vaginal infections within 3 months time.
- After diagnosis and 72 hours of treatment for a vaginal infection, your symptoms continue.
- Vaginal pain occurs during or after sexual intercourse.

YES 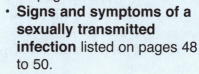 See Provider

NO

Do you have bleeding in the vaginal area from itching due to vaginal irritation? **YES** See Provider

NO

Flowchart continued on next page

Vaginal Problems, *Continued*

Flowchart continued

Do you have vaginal bleeding with any of these problems?
- Increased vaginal bleeding or you continue to have spotting or bleeding between your periods after 3 months of taking birth control pills. (Your dose may need to be adjusted.)
- Bleeding heavier than your normal period (you are saturating almost or equal to 1 full pad or tampon every hour).
- Nausea, vomiting, or abdominal pain.
- Increasing pain and tenderness in your vaginal area.
- Menstrual periods are abnormally heavy or last longer than 10 days.
- You pass many small or large clots with heavy menstrual periods and you are pale and feel very tired.

YES See Provider

NO

Flowchart continued in next column

With vaginal pain, do you use an IUD for birth control and do any of the following conditions apply?
- The IUD was inserted during the last 4 to 6 weeks.
- The strings from the IUD cannot be felt.
- The IUD can be felt through the vagina. (An IUD can become embedded in the wall of the uterus. When this happens, surgery is needed to remove the IUD.)

YES See Provider

NO

Has a vaginal discharge or irritation been present for longer than 1 week despite using Self-Care?

YES 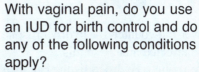 See Provider

NO

 Use Self-Care

Self-Care

For Vaginitis from Contact Dermatitis

- Avoid products that cause the problem (scented items, douches, feminine hygiene sprays, etc.). Don't scrub the affected area with a washcloth.

- Don't wear tight and constricting garments (girdles, tight blue jeans, etc.).

- Use medicated wipes, such as Tucks, instead of dry toilet paper. Follow package directions.

- Add an oatmeal bath product (Aveeno) or baking soda to bath water.

Vaginal Problems, *Continued*

- Apply an over-the-counter 1% hydrocortisone cream to the affected area. Use this infrequently, though. Hydrocortisone can lead to a thinning of the vaginal tissue.

- Put a cool compress on the affected area.

- Take a sitz bath every 4 to 6 hours or as needed. A sitz bath basin is a device that fits on the toilet seat and is used to cleanse the genital area. You can buy a sitz bath basin at a medical supply store and at some drug stores.

- Wash your underwear in a gentle detergent. Rinse it twice. Use only plain water for the second rinse. Don't use fabric softener.

For a Vaginal Yeast Infection

- For a repeat vaginal yeast infection, use an over-the-counter (OTC) vaginal medication, such as Monistat, if it treated the infection successfully in the past. Use it as directed.

{**Note:** Stop using any OTC product for a vaginal yeast infection at least 24 hours before a vaginal exam.}

- Let your health care provider know if you get yeast infections when you take an antibiotic. You may be told to also use an antifungal product.

- Limit sugar and foods with sugar. Sugar promotes the growth of yeast.

- Eat yogurt and/or take an over-the-counter product that contains live cultures of *lactobacillus acidophilus*. Or, take an OTC product that has this.

- Take showers, not baths. Avoid bubble baths.

- Keep the vagina as clean and dry as possible.

- Wear cotton or cotton-lined underwear.

- Don't wear garments that are tight in the crotch. Change underwear and workout clothes right away after you sweat.

- Wear knee-highs instead of panty hose, if possible. When you wear panty hose, wear one with a cotton crotch.

For Information, Contact:

National Women's Health Information Center
800.994.9662 • www.womenshealth.gov

Vomiting & Nausea

"My roommate was real sick. She was throwing up and was real embarrassed because we had a community bathroom. It was pretty gross. But I told her we all get sick."

Tala E., University of Michigan

Signs & Symptoms

- Vomiting is throwing up the stomach's contents. Dry heaves may precede or follow vomiting.

- Nausea is feeling like you're going to vomit.

Causes

- Viruses in the intestines.

- Some medications, such as certain antibiotics.

- Eating too much or eating spoiled food.

- Drinking too much (e.g., alcohol).

- Motion sickness.

- Morning sickness in pregnant females.

Vomiting & Nausea, *Continued*

Medical conditions that cause vomiting include: Labyrinthitis (inflammation of an area in the ear that usually results from an upper respiratory infection); stomach ulcers; hepatitis; meningitis; and a concussion from a head injury. For example, after falling from a loft, dry heaves or vomiting could be a sign of a concussion.

{*Note*: Nausea and vomiting can be signs of having a date rape drug.}

Treatment

Treatment for nausea and/or vomiting depends on the cause.

Questions to Ask

Besides vomiting, do you have **signs and symptoms of meningitis** listed on page 17? **YES** Get Immediate Care

NO

After a recent case of the flu or chicken pox with sudden, repeated vomiting, are other **signs of Reye's Syndrome** listed on page 17 present? **YES** Get Immediate Care

NO

Do dry heaves and/or vomiting occur after a recent head injury or do you vomit true, red blood? **YES** Get Immediate Care

NO

Flowchart continued in next column

With vomiting, are any **signs of alcohol poisoning** listed on page 69 present? **YES** Get Immediate Care

NO

After repeated vomiting, do you have **signs of dehydration** listed on page 24? **YES** Get Immediate Care

NO

With vomiting, do you have **symptoms of an acute kidney infection** listed on page 59? **YES** Get Immediate Care

NO

With nausea or vomiting, do the whites of your eyes or does your skin look yellow? **YES** See Provider

NO

With nausea or vomiting, do you have **symptoms of a bladder infection** listed on page 59? **YES** See Provider

NO

Do you have stomach pain that lasts for more than 2 hours, interferes with your activities, and keeps hurting after you vomit? **YES** See Provider

NO

Flowchart continued on next page

Vomiting & Nausea, *Continued*

Flowchart continued

Do you induce vomiting after overeating or to lose weight? **YES** → **See Provider**

NO ↓

Are you taking medicines that don't work if you vomit, such as asthma medicines? **YES** → **Call Provider**

NO ↓

 Use Self-Care

Self-Care

For Vomiting

- Don't eat solid foods, drink milk or alcohol, smoke, or take aspirin.

- Drink clear liquids, such as water, sport drinks, flat cola and ginger ale. Take small sips. Drink 1 to 2 ounces at a time, but drink often. Suck on ice chips if nothing else will stay down.

- Gradually return to a regular diet, but wait about 8 hours from the last time you vomited. Start with foods that are easy to digest like crackers.

For Nausea Without Vomiting

- Drink clear liquids. Eat small amounts of dry foods, such as soda crackers (if tolerated).

- Avoid things that irritate the stomach, such as alcohol, aspirin, spicy and fried foods.

- For motion sickness, use an over-the-counter antinausea medicine, such as Dramamine. Or use Sea-Bands, a wrist band product that uses acupressure on a certain point on the wrist.

West Nile Virus

Mosquito bites cause West Nile virus if the mosquito is infected with it.

Signs & Symptoms

Most people who get the virus will have no symptoms. About 1 in 5 persons will get mild ones (West Nile fever). Symptoms usually occur 3 to 14 days after being bitten by an infected mosquito. **See Doctor** for the following:

- Fever. Headache. Body aches.

- Skin rash on the trunk of the body (sometimes).

- Swollen lymph glands (sometimes).

About 1 in 150 persons get symptoms of a severe infection (West Nile encephalitis or meningitis). **Get Immediate Care** for the following:

- High fever. Stiff neck. Severe headache. Muscle weakness.

- Tremors. Confusion. Convulsions.

- Decreasing level of consciousness. Paralysis.

Prevention

Protect yourself from mosquito bites. Stay indoors at peak mosquito biting times (dawn, dusk, and early evening). Apply an insect repellent with DEET to clothing and exposed skin to last long enough for the times you will be outdoors. Wear long-sleeved shirts and long pants when you are outdoors.

 For Information, Contact:

Centers for Disease Control and Prevention
www.cdc.gov

CAUTION

General Safety Guidelines

- Learn your school's safety guidelines and follow them. Read your school's safety handbook. Memorize the telephone number(s) for emergency help, such as 9-1-1. Carry a cell phone with you at all times. Pre-program emergency telephone numbers in the phone to be able to call them quickly.

- If you choose to drink, do so responsibly. Don't use drugs. Be careful around other persons who drink heavily and/or use drugs, too. Designate a sober driver.

- Always wear a seatbelt in a motor vehicle. Wear a helmet when riding on a motorcycle, bike, or when rollerblading.

- To avoid being robbed, assaulted, etc.

  - When you go out, go with a friend or a group of people, especially at night and to unfamiliar places.

  - Use ATM machines in well-lit areas, preferably while a friend is with you.

  - Keep your doors and windows locked, especially when you are alone.

  - Lock your bike with a U-shaped lock that is hard for someone to remove.

  - Hold your backpack, purse, etc., securely so someone can't grab it from you. Don't leave these and other personal items, such as your laptop computer, unattended.

  - Have your car, house, or room keys in your hand, ready to unlock your doors.

- If you use social networking Web sites, such as MySpace.com, be aware of potential dangers. Find out safety tips from www.wiredsafety.org.

- Report suspicious behaviors and activities to your school's security or the police.

- Take a class, etc., to learn how to avoid sexual assault.

- To Avoid Fires:

  - Don't smoke in bed or when you are very tired. Better yet, **don't smoke at all!**

  - Follow fire safety precautions when cooking in your dorm room or kitchen.

  - Follow your school's policy on candle use.

  - Keep a working fire extinguisher in your dorm room or house.

- To Manage Conflict Without Violence:

  - Be assertive, not aggressive, when you communicate.

  - Learn to deal with frustration, disappointment, rejection, ridicule, jealousy, and anger.

  - Accept differences in others, including sexual preferences, ethnic and religious backgrounds, etc. You do not need to change your convictions, but don't expect other persons to change their convictions either.

  - Be an active listener. Pay attention to what the other person is saying and try to understand his or her point of view or simply accept it as an opinion.

  - Take a class or seminar in conflict resolution to gain skills in managing conflict.

  - When you can't resolve a conflict on your own, get help.

Playing It Safe

General Safety Guidelines,
Continued

For Information, Contact:

Your school's Student Health Service, Student Counseling or Mental Health Service, Office of Student Conflict Resolution, Office of the Ombudsman, or Student Affairs

The National Crime Prevention Council's Online Resource Center
www.ncpc.org

For Sexual Assault/Hate Crimes/Other Crimes
The National Center for Victims of Crime
www.ncvc.org

National Domestic Violence Hotline
800.799.SAFE (799.7233) • www.ndvh.org

Alcohol & Alcohol Safety

Before drinking, think about its possible consequences (e.g., academic and health problems, unsafe sex, assault, injury, and even death). These consequences affect the person who drinks as well as other students (whether they choose to drink or not) and the community as a whole. See "Effects of Alcohol in Your Blood" box in the next column.

Effects of Alcohol in Your Blood

Alcohol is a central nervous system depressant. How drinking affects your body and mind depends upon your blood alcohol concentration (BAC). BAC is related to how much alcohol you drink in a given period of time and your body weight.

% of Blood Alcohol Concentration (BAC)

Body Weight	Number of Drinks in Two Hours*				
(lbs.)	2	4	6	8	10
120	0.06	0.12	0.19	0.25	0.31
140	0.05	0.11	0.16	0.21	0.27
160	0.05	0.09	0.14	0.19	0.23
180	0.04	0.08	0.13	0.17	0.21
200	0.04	0.08	0.11	0.15	0.19

BAC	Effects
0.05%	Relaxed state. Judgement is not as sharp. Release of tension; carefree feeling.
0.08%**	Inhibitions are lessened.
0.10%	Movements and speech are clumsy.
0.20%	Very drunk. Can be hard to understand. Emotions can be unstable. 100 times greater risk for traffic accident.
0.40%	Deep sleep. Hard to wake up. Not able to make voluntary actions.
0.50%	Can result in coma and/or death.

* 1 drink equals 1½ ounces 80-proof hard liquor, 12 ounces beer, or 5 ounces wine.

** All states use 0.08 as the lowest indicator of driving while intoxicated.

Playing It Safe

Alcohol & Alcohol Safety, *Continued*

Alcohol Poisoning

Call 9-1-1 for one or more of the following signs of alcohol poisoning or combining alcohol and other drugs, such as sedatives or tranquilizers. **Act quickly. Alcohol poisoning can be fatal.**

- Unconsciousness. This means the person is hard to rouse and can't be made aware of his or her surroundings. This can be brief, such as with fainting or blacking out. It can put a person into a coma.

- No breathing or slow and shallow breathing. This means 10 or fewer breaths per minute or time lapses of more than 8 seconds between breaths.

- Slow pulse rate (40 or fewer beats per minute).

- Skin that is cold, clammy, and/or pale or blue in color.

{*Note*: Before emergency care arrives, place the person on his or her side with the knees bent, to prevent choking if he or she vomits. Loosen the person's clothing around the neck and check the mouth and back of the throat to see that nothing obstructs the person's breathing. Stay with the person.}

Alcohol Safety Tips

- Choose substance-free housing, if available and desired.

- Be aware and think about the risks and consequences of drinking, including getting arrested, getting sick, contracting an STI, etc. One incident of alcohol use could cause you to do something you will regret for the rest of your life. Alcohol plays a part in most sexual assaults.

- Mixing drinking with driving, drugs, or operating machines can be fatal. Designate a sober driver.

- Not everyone drinks. Be with people who drink non-alcoholic beverages or ones that look like "drinks," such as non-alcoholic beer in a glass.

- It is better to get medical help for a person who needs it instead of worrying about getting a friend in trouble.

- Drink alcohol only if you want to, and if you do:

  - Know your limit and stick to it or don't drink any alcohol.

  - Drink slowly. You are apt to drink less. Have one drink during a party. Take fake sips, if necessary. In reality, anything over two drinks does not increase the feeling of pleasure. Drinking too much leads to being unable to enjoy yourself.

  - Eat when you drink. Food helps to slow alcohol absorption.

  - Alternate an alcoholic beverage with a non-alcoholic one. Use non-alcohol or reduced alcohol beverages. Dilute distilled beverages. Use more and more mixer and less and less alcohol. After two drinks, your taste buds are dulled and you won't be able to notice much difference.

  - Avoid drinking contests and games.

Playing It Safe

Alcohol & Alcohol Safety, *Continued*

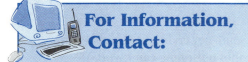

For Information, Contact:

Emergency Medical Service (Call 9-1-1) if you suspect alcohol poisoning or a drug overdose

Your school's Student Health Service, Student Counseling Service, or Alcohol and other Drug Program

Al-Anon/Alateen World Service Office
888.4AL.ANON (425.2666) • www.al-anon.org

Alcoholics Anonymous (AA) World Services
www.aa.org

Center for Substance Abuse Treatment (CSAT)
National Drug Treatment Referral Routing Service
800.662.HELP (4357)
www.findtreatment.samhsa.gov

Narcotics Anonymous (NA)
818.773.9999 • www.na.org

National Institute on Alcohol Abuse & Alcoholism (NIAAA)
www.niaaa.nih.gov • www.thecoolspot.gov

Drugs & Drug Safety

After alcohol, the most common drugs used on college campuses are tobacco (see "**Tobacco Use – Benefits of Quitting**" on page 88) and marijuana. Other drugs used are amphetamines (uppers); barbiturates (downers); hallucinogens, such as LSD; inhalants; and narcotics, such as cocaine. On the increase is the use of substances known collectively as "club drugs." These are used at all-night dance parties, such as "raves" or "trances," dance clubs, and bars. Examples are MDMA (Ecstasy), GHB, Rohypnol, Ketamine, methamphetamine, and LSD.

The safest use of drugs is <u>no use</u> of drugs!

Drug Chart	
Drug Name(s)	**Dangers of Use**
Cocaine. This drug is also called blow, crack, crank, "C", coke, nose candy, rock, and white girl.	Increases pulse rate and blood pressure. Causes insomnia, irritability, and paranoia. Can result in severe depression, convulsions, heart attack, lung damage, hallucinations, brain damage, risk of infection (hepatitis, HIV from using contaminated needles), coma, and death.

Chart continued on the next page

Playing It Safe

Drugs & Drug Safety, *Continued*

Chart continued

Drug Name(s)	Dangers of Use
Depressants. Examples are alcohol, barbiturates, sedatives, tranquilizers, downers, ludes, reds, and yellow jackets.	Causes drowsiness, slurred speech, drunkenness, memory loss, sudden mood shifts, depression, and lack of coordination. Can result in shallow breathing, dilated pupils, clammy skin, weak pulse, coma, and death.
Ecstasy. This is MDMA. Other names are Adam, Clarity, Lover's Speed, and K.	Euphoric state initially, but depression can occur after taking the drug. Also carries the risk of a heat stroke from lack of fluids and sweating from dancing too long, especially in the hot environment of a club. May lead to a heart attack, seizure, and stroke.
GHB and GLB (a similar drug that turns into GHB in the body). Other names are: Grievous Bodily Harm; Liquid Ecstacy, Liquid Sex, Georgia Home Boy, and Scoop.	Common date rape drug that results in nausea, vomiting, a feeling of intoxication, and amnesia-like symptoms. The drug slows the heartbeat, reduces blood pressure, and can cause the user's breathing to stop. Overdose results in unconsciousness, coma, and eventual death. There is little difference in the dose that can get someone high and one that can cause death.
Inhalants. Examples are vapors from: Solvents, such as gasoline; aerosols, such as hair sprays; anesthetics, such as ether, chloroform, nitrous oxide; and spray paints, especially gold and silver.	Slows heart rate, breathing and brain activity. Can cause headaches, dizziness, nausea, lack of coordination, slurred speech, blurred vision. Can result in suffocation, heart failure, unconsciousness, seizures, brain damage, and even death.
Ketamine. This drug is also called: Special K, K, Vitamin K, and Cat Valium.	Causes dream-like states and hallucinations. Can cause delirium, amnesia, impaired motor functions, high blood pressure, depression, and breathing problems that can result in death.
LSD. This is also called acid, bloomers, and yellow sunshines.	Causes hallucinations, dilated pupils, increased heart rate and blood pressure, sweating, sleeplessness, dry mouth, and tremors. Nausea, weakness, numbness or trembling are common. Long term use can cause persistent psychosis and what used to be called "flashbacks" – re-experiencing symptoms of past hallucinogen use even though not taking the drug at the present time.

Chart continued on the next page

 To Learn More, See Back Cover

Playing It Safe

Drugs & Drug Safety, *Continued*

Chart continued

Drug Name(s)	Dangers of Use
Marijuana. This is also called pot, grass, reefer, herb, jay, joint, smoke, weed, and AMP (marijuana with formaldehyde).	Can result in feelings of panic, impaired short term memory, decreased ability to concentrate, fatigue, paranoia, and possible psychosis. Also causes lung damage. Synthetic marijuana, such as K2 can have serious side effects, such as extremely high blood pressure, very fast heartbeat, paranoia, delusions, seizure, and hallucinations.
Methamphetamine. This drug is also called speed, ice, chalk, crystal meth, crack, fire, and glass.	Can result in memory loss, agitation, aggression, and violent or psychotic behavior and potential cardiac and neurological damage. Can contribute to higher rates of transmission of hepatitis and HIV, if injected. Can result in heart attacks, seizures, and death from overdose.
Rohypnol. This is also called R-2, Rib, Roofies, Rope, and Forget-Me Pill.	Common date rape drug. Used in sexual assaults. Results in decreased blood pressure, drowsiness, visual disturbances, confusion, nausea, and vomiting. When mixed with alcohol or other drugs, this clear, odorless, and tasteless drug can cause death.

Signs of a Drug Overdose

Signs of an overdose depend on the type of drug used. Call 9-1-1 or get emergency care for one or more of the following:

- Unconsciousness. This means the person is hard to rouse and can't be made aware of his or her surroundings. This can be brief, such as with fainting or blacking out. It can put a person into a coma.

- No breathing or slow and shallow breathing. This means 10 or fewer breaths per minute or time lapses of more than 8 seconds between breaths.

- Slow pulse rate (40 or fewer beats per minute).

- Suicidal gestures.

- Seizures.

- Tremors.

- Sudden hostile personality or violent behavior.

- Very rapid pulse rate (140 or more beats per minute) and/or extreme anxiety or paranoia.

For Information, Contact: Places listed on page 70.

Drugs & Drug Safety, *Continued*

Penalties for Drug Use

Be aware of the penalties your school and law enforcement authorities can and will take if you possess, use, make, and/or distribute alcohol or illicit drugs. Penalties vary, based on your school's policy and on the laws that govern certain substances. Penalties your school may take range from verbal or written reprimands to suspension or expulsion from the school. You can be fined and/or put in prison for prosecution of a misdemeanor or felony, depending on the nature of the offense. For example, conviction of possessing or using cocaine, heroin, or even GHB, could put you in prison for up to 20 years. If you give GHB to someone else and that person dies, you could be convicted of manslaughter. If you are of legal drinking age and give alcohol to a minor and it causes death, you could be convicted of a felony that carries a 10 year prison sentence.

Over-the-Counter Medication Safety

- Read warning sections on labels or look up the name of the medicine in the *Physician's Desk Reference for Nonprescription Drugs*. If you are unsure about taking an over-the-counter (OTC) medicine, check with your health care provider or pharmacist. Find out if it is safe to combine medicines (prescribed or OTC ones), to take alcohol with a medicine, or to take OTC herbs, such as kava kava and St. John's Wort with medicines and/or alcohol.

- Before you take a medicine, check the expiration date. Discard ones that have expired.

- Know what medications you are allergic to. Check the labels on all OTC medicines to see if what you are allergic to is in them. Also, wear a medical alert tag to let others know about allergies to medications as well as medical conditions you have. Get a medical alert tag from a drugstore or from MedicAlert Foundation International, 800.344.3226, www.medicalert.org.

- Do not take OTC medicines on a regular basis unless your health care provider tells you to.

- Don't take someone else's prescribed medicines. Don't take OTC medicines that you are not familiar with or are not in the original product package. Don't give your prescribed medicine to others.

- Follow directions on the medicine's label. Do not exceed the dose(s) specified. For example, if you take 2 acetaminophen (e.g., Tylenol) tablets for a headache, don't take 2 more in 2 hours if the label instructs you to take 2 tablets every 4 to 6 hours. Also, don't take another pain reliever, such as ibuprofen (e.g., Advil) or a medicine with acetaminophen, such as Nyquil, at the same time or within the same 4 hours of taking acetaminophen. This is too much medicine.

- If you are under 19 years of age, do not take aspirin or any medicines that contain salicylates, such as Pepto Bismol, due to its link to Reye's Syndrome. This is especially true when you have the flu or chicken pox.

- If you order prescriptions and OTC medications online, make sure that a registered pharmacist checks for drug interactions. Access www.nabp.net for a location that the National Association of Boards of Pharmacy has given a verified Internet Pharmacy Practice Site (VIPDS) seal of approval.

Playing It Safe

Over-the-Counter Medication Safety, *Continued*

Basic Over-the-Counter (OTC) Medications		
Medicines	**Common Uses**	**Side Effects/Warnings/Interactions**
Antacids (e.g., Tums, Rolaids, Mylanta).	Stomach upset. Heartburn.	Don't use for more than 2 weeks without your doctor's advice. Don't use high-sodium ones if on a low-salt diet. Don't use if you have chronic kidney failure.
Antidiarrheal medicine (e.g., Kaopectate, Imodium A-D, Pepto-Bismol).	Diarrhea.	Don't give Pepto-Bismol to anyone under 19 years of age. It contains salicylates, which have been linked to Reye's Syndrome. Also, Pepto-Bismol can cause black stools.
Antihistamines (e.g., Chlor-Trimeton, Benadryl).	Allergies. Cold symptom relief. Relieves itching.	May make you drowsy or agitated. Can cause dry mouth and/or problems with urinating. Don't use with alcohol, when operating machines, or when driving. Don't use if you have glaucoma or an enlarged prostate or problems passing urine.
Cough suppressant (e.g., Robitussin-DM or others with dextromethorphan).	Dry cough without mucus.	May make you drowsy. If taken in large quantities (10-30 times the recommended dose): can result in euphoria and a feeling of being disconnected; can cause blackouts, delusions, dizziness, heart palpitations, insomnia, or seizures; coma or death can occur.
Decongestant (e.g., Sudafed, Dimetapp).	Stuffy and runny nose. Postnasal drip. Allergies. Fluid in the ears.	Don't use if you have high blood pressure, diabetes, glaucoma, heart disease, a history of stroke, or an enlarged prostate.
Expectorant (e.g., Robitussin or others with guaifenesin).	Cough with mucus.	Don't give with an antihistamine.
Laxatives (e.g., Ex-Lax, Correctol (stimulant-types), Metamucil (bulk-forming type).	Constipation.	Long-term use of stimulant-type can lead to dependence and to muscle weakness due to potassium loss.
Throat anesthetic (e.g., Sucrets, Chloraseptic spray).	Minor sore throat.	Don't give throat lozenges to children under age 5.
Toothache anesthetic (e.g., Anbesol).	Toothache. Teething.	Call doctor before giving to babies under 4 months old.

Chart continued on the next page

Playing It Safe

Over-the-Counter Medication Safety, *Continued*

Medicines	Common Uses	Side Effects/Warnings/Interactions
Pain Relievers		
Acetaminophen (e.g., Tylenol, Anacin-3, Datril, Liquiprin, Panadol, Tempra).	Gives pain relief. Lowers fever. Does not reduce swelling.	More gentle on stomach than other OTC pain relievers. Can result in liver problems in heavy alcohol users. Large doses or long-term use can cause liver or kidney damage.
Aspirin* (e.g., Bayer, Bufferin).	Gives pain relief. Lowers fever and swelling.	Can cause stomach upset (which is made worse with alcohol use). May cause stomach ulcers and bleeding. Avoid if you: Have an ulcer, have asthma, are under 19 years of age (due to its link to Reye's Syndrome), and/or are having surgery within 2 weeks. High doses or prolonged use can cause ringing in the ears.
Ibuprofen* (e.g., Advil, Motrin, Adult and Children's Advil). **Ketoprofen*** for adults (e.g., Actron, Orudis KT). **Naproxen Sodium*** for adults (e.g., Aleve).	Gives pain relief. Lowers fever and swelling.	Can cause stomach upset and peptic ulcers. Take with milk or food. Can make you more sensitive to the effects of the sun. Don't use if you are allergic to aspirin. Don't use if you have a peptic ulcer, blood clotting problems, or kidney disease.

* These medicines are examples of nonsteroidal anti-inflammatory drugs (NSAIDs).

{*Note:* Consult your health care provider about using herbal products and nutritional supplements. Harm can result from the product itself, taking too much of it, and/or combining it with other products, including OTC and prescription medicines. <u>DO</u> <u>NOT</u> take: Anabolic steroids; muscle building products, Green Hornet, Liquid Speed, Snuffadelic, or Adderrall (to pull an all nighter). These can cause major health problems. So can Ritalin. Take this only if and as prescribed by your health care provider.}

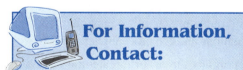

For Information, Contact:

Food and Drug Administration
www.fda.gov

National Center for Complementary and Alternative Medicine (NCCAM)
888.644.6226 • www.nccam.nih.gov

 To Learn More, See Back Cover

Playing It Safe

Dealing with Traumatic Events

The mass shootings at Columbine High School in 1999 and at Virginia Tech University in 2007 have heightened awareness that traumatic events can occur on school campuses. These events can have an impact on people who have seen them first hand and people who have witnessed the events on television or the Internet. As one student said, "It's scary because situations like this make you realize how vulnerable you really are."

Read common blogs and it is clear to see that incidents like these prompt the following questions:

- How could this have happened?
- Why wasn't this prevented?
- How can this be prevented in the future?
- How can I protect myself?

The last question is, perhaps the most important one for students and parents. What can you do to protect yourself? Here are some suggestions:

- Be alert and aware of what's going on around you.
- Find out your school's policy on crisis situations and the procedures to follow.
- Report any threats or threatening behaviors to the appropriate person or department established by your school. Know who to contact ahead of time. Program the number in your cell phone. Find out if information you give is kept confidential, if this is an issue for you.
- If you witness an emergency situation, call campus police or 9-1-1!

Other Traumatic Events

Natural disasters, such as hurricanes, floods, and tornados, can also be catastrophic for students, teachers, parents, and the communities they affect. Also, an event does not have to reach the proportions of a hurricane or campus shooting to be a traumatic one. It can be any event or series of events that cause a lot of stress for an individual. Examples are losing a loved one, being injured, and being rejected.

A traumatic event is marked by a sense of helplessness, horror, serious injury, or the threat of serious injury or death. It affects the person who survives it, as well as his or her friends and relatives.

Common Responses to a Traumatic Event

Physical Responses

- Crying. Feeling numb.
- Inability to rest. Sleep problems.
- Changes in appetite.
- Exhaustion.
- The need to be comforted and to give comfort.
- Increased heart rate.
- Easily startled. Hyper-vigilance.
- Withdrawal from normal activities.
- Headache and other body aches and pains.

Emotional Reactions

- Anger. Blaming others.
- Anxiety. Depression.
- Guilt. Feeling helpless and hopeless.
- Fear. Flashbacks. Nightmares.
- Feeling "unreal" as if everything is a dream.

Dealing with Traumatic Events, *Continued*

Ways to Help Cope with Traumatic Events

- Know that your symptoms are normal, especially right after the traumatic event.

- Give yourself time to heal. Know that this may not be an easy time. Allow yourself to feel whatever you are feeling. Be patient with changes in your feelings.

- If you are physically able, start doing strenuous activity within the first 72 hours of the event. Alternate physical exercise with relaxation.

- Maintain good health habits. Eat healthy foods. Plan for enough sleep.

- Keep to your normal routine as much as you can. Keep busy. Focus on class assignments, campus activities, work, etc.

- Try not to isolate yourself. Connect with people. Visit, call, or send text messages to people who will support you. Rely on friends, teachers, family, and support groups. It can be comforting to talk to persons who have experienced the same or similar event.

- Accept the fact that some things are out of your control.

- Express your feelings in a journal, poetry, drawings, etc.

- Accept the kindness of others.

- Help others in need. Doing this is a way to take the focus off yourself and to manage your own feelings.

Most people report feeling better within a few months after a traumatic event. When the following symptoms begin within 6 weeks to 3 months after the event and **last for at least 1 month**, a person experiencing them may have posttraumatic stress disorder (PTSD). If you experience these symptoms or suspect someone you know does, contact your school's Student Health Service, Student Counseling Service or a health care provider.

Signs & Symptoms of PTSD

"Avoidance Symptoms"

Avoiding people, places, and activities that recall the event.

Avoiding thoughts, feelings, or mention of the event.

Having much less interest in doing necessary activities.

Feeling detached or estranged from others.

Forgetting an important aspect of the event.

"Increased Arousal" Symptoms

Being very easily startled.

Having a hard time concentrating.

Having a hard time falling or staying asleep.

Being very cranky.

"Re-living" the Event Symptoms

Having recurring, intrusive thoughts of the event that cause distress.

Having flashbacks of the event.

Having nightmares.

Treatment

Posttraumatic stress disorder, in most cases, should be treated by a mental health professional. Treatment can usually be done on an outpatient basis.

Playing It Safe

Skin Safety

The skin is your body's largest organ. It protects your internal organs from environmental irritants, infections, and ultraviolet light; all of which can be harmful. Take good care of your skin so it can do its job. Keep your skin clean and protect it from injury. (See "**Skin Injuries**" on page 38.)

Protect Your Skin From Sun Damage

Do you look forward to semester breaks so you can relax in the sun and get a tan? Many students do. A suntan looks good, but it is a sign that your skin is trying to protect itself from damage. Be especially careful not to get sunburned. In fact, you should never get sunburned! It can lead to premature aging, wrinkling of the skin, and skin cancer. (Be extra cautious if you have a family history of skin cancer.) Even if you are not concerned about these problems now, the pain and blisters that come with a severe sunburn can make spring break unbearable.

The risk for sunburn is increased for persons with fair skin, blue eyes, red or blond hair, and for persons taking some medicines. These include birth control pills; some antibiotics, such as tetracycline and sulfa drugs; and Benadryl, an over-the-counter antihistamine.

To Prevent Sunburn

- Avoid exposure to the midday sun (10 a.m. to 4 p.m. standard time or 11 a.m. to 5 p.m. daylight saving time).

- Use sunscreen with a sun protection factor (SPF) of 15 to 30 or more when exposed to the sun. The lighter your skin, the higher the SPF number should be. Apply the sunscreen 15 to 30 minutes before you go out in the sun.

Use about 2 tablespoons to adequately cover all exposed body parts. Reapply sunscreen every 60 to 90 minutes, even if the sunscreen is water-resistant.

- Along with sunscreen, use moisturizers, makeup, lip balm, etc. that contain sunscreen. Use water-based ones if you have acne.

- Wear a wide-brimmed hat and long sleeves.

- Wear clothing with sunscreen protection or muted colors, such as tan. Bright colors and white reflect the sun onto the face.

- Wear sunglasses that absorb at least 90% of both UVA and UVB rays.

Tattoo and Body Piercing Safety

You may already have one or more tattoos and/or area(s) of your body pierced. You may be thinking about getting one of these procedures done as a way to fit in and look like others; as a way to express your individuality; and/or to get noticed. Before you get a tattoo or a part of your body pierced, consider the following:

- In many states, the law does not allow minors to get tattoos. Find out about this in your state.

- Unsterile tattooing equipment and needles can transmit serious infectious diseases, such as tetanus, hepatitis B, and HIV. Never do one of these procedures on yourself or have anyone else do it that is not certified by the Association of Professional Piercers (APP) or the Alliance of Professional Tattooists (APT). Certified members are trained in strict safety and health requirements. Because of the high risk of infection, you cannot donate blood for one year after getting a tattoo.

Skin Safety, *Continued*

■ Tattoos and body piercings also carry the risk of less serious local infections. You will need to follow proper care procedures for weeks or months after the procedure to reduce the risk of getting an infection. You may also get large growths of scar tissues called keloids.

■ Tattoos are not easily removed and in some cases may cause permanent discoloration. Keep a record of the dyes used in the tattoo you get. This includes the lot number of each pigment. If you choose to get a tattoo removed in the future, this information will be helpful. Think carefully before getting a tattoo and consider the possibility of an allergic reaction. Know that it is expensive, too, to get a tattoo removed. Don't get a tattoo or body piercing done on an impulse. Wait at least 24 hours. In the meantime, read about the things to consider in this topic and see "**For Information, Contact**" places on this page. Also, ask your friends who have tattoos and/or body piercings about their experiences. Find out about the pain involved, the healing time, the cost, etc.

■ Visit several tattoo parlors to see whether the tattooist follows recommended safety guidelines and sterilization techniques, such as using a heat sterilization machine regulated by the Food and Drug Administration (FDA).

■ According to the APT guidelines, these practices should be followed:

• The tattooist should have an autoclave (a heat sterilization machine regulated by the FDA) on the premises.

• Consent forms (which the customer must sign) should be handed out before tattooing.

• Immediately before tattooing, the tattooist should wash and dry his or her hands thoroughly and put on medical latex gloves, which should be worn at all times during application of the tattoo.

• Needle bars and tubes should be autoclaved after each customer. Non-autoclavable surfaces, such as pigment bottles, drawer pulls, chairs, tables, sinks, and the immediate floor area, should be cleaned with a disinfectant, such as a bleach solution.

• Used absorbent tissues should be placed in a special puncture-resistant, leak-proof container for disposal.

■ For body piercing, to avoid allergic reactions and infections, jewelry made from non-corrosive, non-toxic metals should be used. Examples are solid 14K gold (not gold-plated), niobium, surgical stainless steel, and titanium.

■ After the procedure, follow the skin care guidelines provided by your skin piercer or tattooist. Care of the site will depend on its location and/or the procedure you had done.

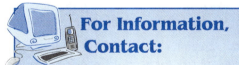

For Information, Contact:

For Sun Safety
National Cancer Institute
800.4.CANCER (422.6237)
www.cancer.gov

Playing It Safe

Tests & Immunizations

Tests

The following tests are general recommendations for persons between the ages of 11 and 26. If you have an increased risk for certain conditions, testing may need to be done sooner or more often. Additional tests may also be needed. Follow your doctor's or health care provider's advice for health tests and exams. You can get updates and more information on screening tests and exams from healthfinder.gov at www.healthfinder.gov/myhealthfinder.

Health Test	Ages 11–18	Ages 19–26
Height & Weight	Every year or as advised by health care provider	
Regular Dental Checkup	Every 6 months or at least every year	
Blood Pressure	During office visits	During office visits or at least every 2 years
Chlamydia Screening[1]	All sexually active females aged 25 and younger	
HIV Screeing	All persons ages 15-65 should be screened for HIV	
Pap Test (Females)	At least every 3 years starting at age 21	
Cholesterol Blood Test[2]		As advised by your health care provider

1. Screening is also recommended for females older than age 25 who: Have more than one sexual partner; have had an STI in the past; or who do not use condoms consistently and correctly. After initial screening, follow your health care provider's advice for how often to have re-screenings.

2. In general, screening tests for blood cholesterol should begin at age 35 for men and age 45 for women at an increased risk for heart disease. You may need to begin screening tests sooner if you have diabetes, high blood pressure, or a family history of heart disease.

Playing It Safe

Tests & Immunizations, *Continued*

Immunizations

This chart shows vaccine guidelines for persons ages 11 to 26, provided recommended childhood vaccines have already been received. Guidelines may change. For more information and updates on vaccines, contact your doctor or healthcare provider and the Centers for Disease Control and Prevention (CDC) at www.cdc.gov/vaccines.

Vaccine	Recommendation
Influenza (Flu)	Yearly seasonal flu vaccine. Follow health care provider's advice for other types of flu vaccines, if any.
Tdap (Tetanus, Diphtheria, Acellular Pertussis) Td (Tetanus/Diphtheria)	Age 11-12 years or at age 13 through 18 years, if not previously vaccinated, or a one-time dose as an adult. After that, a Td booster should be given every 10 years.
Human Papillomavirus (HPV)	Age 11-12 years, but can be given from age 9 through 26 years. Three doses can prevent the most common type of HPV that can cause cervical cancer and genital warts.
Meningococcal (MCV4)	Age 11-12 years or at age 13 through 18 years, if not previously vaccinated. May be required for unvaccinated college freshmen who live in dorms.
Measles, Mumps, Rubella (MMR)	Two doses by age 18 years. Your school may require proof of immunity or vaccination.
Hepatitis B	A 3-dose series should be given to children, teenagers, and high risk adults who have not yet had 3 doses of this vaccine.
Varicella (Chicken Pox)	Two doses for persons who have not had chicken pox or who have not yet had 2 doses of this vaccine.

Also, before you travel to other countries, find out if you need certain vaccines. Do this several months before you plan to travel to allow enough time to get required vaccines. Get information from 800.CDC.INFO (232.4636) or at www.cdc.gov/travel. Discuss your needs with your healthcare provider.

Testicular Self-Exam (TSE)

Cancer of the testicles, the primary male sex glands, is the most common type of cancer in males aged 15 to 35.

Starting at age 15, talk to your doctor or health care provider about doing testicular self-exams (TSEs). If you choose to do TSEs, do them as advised.

The best time to do a TSE is after a warm shower or bath. This relaxes the scrotum, allows the testicles to drop down, and makes it easier to find anything unusual.

Doing a TSE is easy and takes only a few minutes.

1. Stand in front of a mirror. Look for any swelling on the skin of the scrotum.

2. Examine each testicle with both hands. Place your index and middle fingers underneath the testicle and your 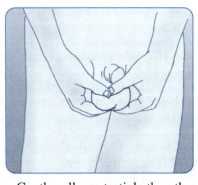 thumbs on top. Gently roll one testicle then the other between your thumbs and fingers. One testicle may be larger. This is normal. Examine for any lumps. (These are usually painless and about the size of a pea (lump)).

3. Find the epididymis (the comma-shaped cord behind the testicle). This may be tender to the touch. Examine it for lumps.

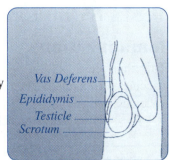

Vas Deferens
Epididymis
Testicle
Scrotum

4. Examine the vas deferens (the tubelike structure at the back of each testicle) for lumps.

Reasons to Contact Your Health Care Provider

- A lump on a testicle, epididymis, or vas deferens.

- An enlarged testicle.

- A heavy feeling, pain, or discomfort in the testicle or scrotum or a change in the way the testicle feels.

- A dull ache in the lower abdomen or the groin.

- A sudden collection of fluid in the scrotum.

- Enlarged or tender breasts.

These can be signs of cancer or another condition, such as an infection. When found early, testicular cancer is very curable.

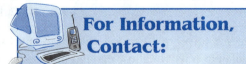

For Information, Contact:

Cancer Information Service
800.4.CANCER (422.6237) • www.cancer.gov

The Testicular Cancer Resource Center
www.acor.org

Playing It Safe

Breast Awareness & Self-Exam (BSE)

How To Do a BSE

Breast awareness is knowing how your breasts normally look and feel and checking for changes. You can do this while you shower or get dressed. A breast self-exam (BSE) is a step-by-step method to examine your breasts. Beginning at age 20, ask your health care provider about the pros and cons of doing a BSE. If you choose to do a BSE, examine your breasts during times of the month when they are not normally tender or swollen. If you menstruate, the best time may be within 3 days after your period stops.

BSE Steps

1. Lie down:
Place a pillow under your right shoulder. Put your right hand behind your head. Move the

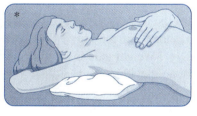

pads of your left hand's 3 middle fingers, held flat, in small, circular motions as you start to feel your right breast tissue. Use this circular motion in an up and down pattern as you check the entire breast area. This includes the area from as high up as your collarbone to as low as the ribs below your breast; and from your right side (from under your arm) across the breast to the middle of your chest bone. Feel every part of this entire area with 3 different levels of pressure:

- Light – Feel the tissue closest to the skin.
- Medium – Feel a little deeper than the skin.
- Firm– Feel the tissue closest to your chest and ribs.

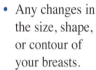

2. Squeeze the nipple gently. Check for a clear or bloody discharge.

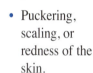

3. Repeat steps 1 and 2 for the left breast using the finger pads of your right hand.

4. Stand in front of a mirror. Press your hands firmly on your hips. Look for:

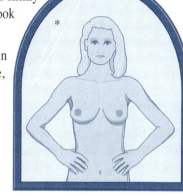

- Any changes in the size, shape, or contour of your breasts.

- Puckering, scaling, or redness of the skin.

- Nipple changes or discharge.

5. Sit or stand. Raise your arm slightly. Examine each underarm area for lumps or changes.

If you a find a lump or any change in the way your breasts normally look or feel, let your health care provider know right away. Most lumps that are found and tested are not cancer.

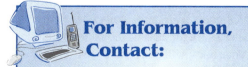

For Information, Contact:

The National Cancer Institute
800.4.CANCER (422.6237) • www.cancer.gov

Playing It Safe

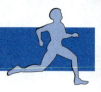

Eat Well & Get Regular Exercise

Here you are at college. Maybe this is the first time you have lived on your own. Are you wondering what to eat? Worried about gaining weight? Concerned about looking good and staying fit? The food and exercise choices you make will play a major role in helping you not only stay healthy, but also increase your ability to do well in classes.

A Few Words About the Basics

Much like a car, your body runs best when supplied with the most efficient source of fuel, in this case – carbohydrates. Carbohydrates are classified as either simple or complex. Simple carbohydrates, often called sugars, occur naturally in some foods, especially fruits. Complex carbohydrates, commonly known as starches, are found in grains (rice, bread, pasta), beans, and vegetables, particularly starchy vegetables, such as potatoes and corn.

Frequently accused as fattening, carbohydrates are actually very filling and help you maintain a healthy weight. Carbohydrates contain four calories per gram; fats have 9. It would take a man who needs 3,000 calories 30 potatoes to maintain his body weight if no other foods were eaten!

Carbohydrates are not as easily turned into body fat as are dietary fats because they "burn" more efficiently. Of course, any time you consistently eat more calories (regardless of the source) than you burn, your body will store the excess energy as fat. The guideline is to eat about 55 to 60% of your calories from carbohydrates, primarily complex ones. A good way to visualize this is to have carbohydrate foods occupy two-thirds of the food on your plate.

Fats add flavor to foods and also help you feel full from a meal. Although fat is one of the most criticized nutrients, some fat in the diet is necessary because it supplies essential fatty acids. The guideline is to eat 30% or less of your calories from fats. This is about 60 to 65 grams of fat per day for the average person.

How about protein? Protein is found in both animal and plant sources and is an essential nutrient for it is the main structural component of all tissues in the body. The guideline is to eat 10 to 15% of your calories from protein. This amount is easily supplied from foods you eat. Excessive intake of protein (whether from foods or supplements) may actually create health problems and does not lead to greater muscle mass!

Weight Worries

Has the fear of "The Freshman Fifteen" set in yet? Weight gain is not an inevitable part of college life. Sometimes, weight 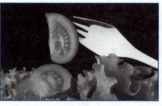 gain is even acceptable. Cafeteria meals, fast food, and regular restaurants all offer a variety of healthy food choices. Strive for a balance. If you choose a higher calorie food, such as french fries with a meal, balance it with lower calorie items – vegetables, salad with low-fat dressing, and fresh fruit.

Want to know more about balancing your diet and weight? Check out the information available through the Web sites listed on page 86. Or, browse in your bookstore for The American Dietetic Association's Complete Food and Nutrition Guide by Roberta Duyff or Dieting for Dummies by Jane Kirby.

Lifestyle Issues

Eat Well & Get Regular Exercise, *Continued*

Don't forget the other side of the equation which is exercise. Eating right and exercising regularly will keep you in top form. Do exercises that you enjoy. Exercise at least 3 times a week. Choose some form of aerobic exercise, such as walking, swimming, Tai (Tae) Bo, etc. Do stretching and strengthening exercises, too. For more information on exercise, access the Web site: www.fitness.gov.

Breakfast for Better Grades

Starting the day with breakfast is the key to learning. People who eat breakfast perform better on cognitive tests, have better verbal fluency, and increased memory. This may not translate into passing college chemistry, but it does give you a fighting chance.

Eating breakfast also helps you maintain weight. People who eat breakfast generally burn 4 to 6% more calories than people who do not eat breakfast.

Many students skip breakfast. It is best if you don't. For breakfast, have whole grain cereal and milk; a breakfast sandwich on whole grain bread; yogurt with granola; cottage cheese with fresh fruit; leftover pizza, or a muffin or bagel with milk and an apple. Take a bagel or pop tart and a juice box to class with you, if you don't set aside time to eat breakfast.

Going Vegetarian?

If you are thinking about trying a vegetarian eating style, you may not know where to begin. Vegetarianism means eating mostly plant foods. If you include dairy and egg products in your eating plan, it is easier to meet your nutrient needs. If you're a vegan – which means you only eat plant foods – you may need to supplement your diet with calcium, iron, zinc, and vitamins B_{12} and D.

Start slowly. Begin by changing some of your favorite recipes – decrease meat and add more pasta, beans, rice, or vegetables. Look for vegetarian meat alternatives, like soy or veggie burgers. Experiment with different types of beans, pasta, and rice. Try red, black, navy, or pinto beans, or split peas and lentils. Look for different types of rice – from plain white to mixed brown and long grain. Top salads with chickpeas or red beans instead of cheese. You will also need to increase fluids, such as water or juices, to help with the increased fiber.

If you are looking for more information on being a vegetarian, try www.vrg.org (The Vegetarian Resource Group).

Snacks and Your Backpack

Snacking is a big part of hectic college life. When you are out shopping for snacks, stock up on pretzels, fruit, graham crackers, mini-size cereal boxes, popcorn, meal replacement bars, etc.

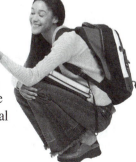

Lifestyle Issues

Eat Well & Get Regular Exercise, *Continued*

If snacking and studying go together, try setting a schedule. Study for one hour and then grab a snack. This helps keep calories in control. Measure out a portion size of the snack rather than eating out of a large box or bag.

When it comes to eating on the run, have a 6 inch submarine sandwich on a whole grain roll or a vegetarian pita. Don't go long periods of time without eating. This leaves you famished and fatigued.

Stress and Emotional Eating

College life may leave you feeling stressed. Do you need extra vitamins and nutrients? Though a busy schedule may sometimes cause people to neglect eating well, we do not use any more (or fewer) nutrients while under mental stress. When you are feeling stressed and strung-out, try these tips:

- Take time to take care of yourself. This includes taking time to eat well. Don't just snack all day. Sit down and enjoy your meal.

- Try quick foods, such as fresh, canned, or frozen veggies added to canned soups or pastas. Order in if you like, but try not to skip meals.

- Start your day with breakfast! It will help you get going for the rest of the day.

Food cravings may be a sign of hunger created from skipping meals, from a lack of nutrients in your diet, or an attempt to satisfy emotional needs. Food won't solve your emotional dilemmas. The next time you find yourself heading for the fridge for a quick emotional fix, use the tips in the next column.

- You are studying for that big exam and find yourself nervous and anxious. Instead of splurging on ice cream, seek out different relaxation techniques. Sit quietly with your eyes closed and breathe deeply for a few minutes. Or, go for a quick walk. Get enough sleep. Sleep deprivation makes most people anxious and irritable.

- You've had a big fight with your roommate and are furious. Anger can cause overeating quicker than most other emotions. Instead of eating as a response to this, try, instead, to confront the target of your anger. Have that difficult conversation after you have had a chance to calm down or write out your feelings in a letter.

- You find yourself with nothing to do, but sit around and eat. Many people eat out of boredom. Solution? Diversion! Find something else to capture your attention. Find which diversions work best for you and use them.

- Most importantly, don't spend time feeling guilty when you eat to get an emotional fix. Doing this occasionally is not a problem.

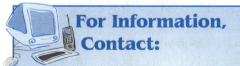

For Information, Contact:

ChooseMyPlate.gov
www.choosemyplate.gov/MyPlateonCampus

Go Ask Alice Web site
www.goaskalice.columbia.edu

Set Up Good Sleep Habits

- Plan ahead. Don't start writing a paper the night before it is due or cram for a test the night before you have it. Doing these things starts a cycle of staying up all night and never catching up on sleep.

- Get at least 30 minutes of sunlight exposure daily.

- Get regular exercise, but not within a few hours of going to bed.

- If you have a roommate, discuss and decide when your room will be used for studying, socializing, and sleep.

- If your dorm is too noisy to sleep, talk to your resident advisor and/or learn to tune out the noise in order to get to sleep. If it helps, listen to soft music with earphones when you fall asleep. Wear earplugs, if necessary.

- Make your dorm room or bedroom as comfortable as possible. Create a quiet, dark atmosphere. Keep the room temperature comfortable (neither too warm nor too cold). Don't wait longer than a week to change the sheets on your bed.

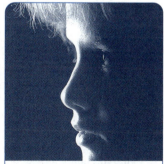

An hour or two before going to bed, dim the lights in your room.

- Have food items rich in the amino acid L-tryptophan, such as milk, turkey, or tuna fish, before you go to bed. Eating foods with carbohydrates, such as cereal, breads, and fruits may help as well. (Do not, however, take L-tryptophan supplements.)

- Develop a regular bedtime routine. Brush your teeth, lock or check doors and windows, get your backpack ready for the next day, etc. Try to go to bed and get up at the same time every day.

- Take a long, warm bath or shower before bedtime.

- Read a book or do some repetitive, calm activity. Avoid distractions that may hold your attention and keep you awake, such as watching a suspenseful movie.

- Avoid caffeine in all forms after lunchtime. Caffeine is in coffee, tea, chocolate, colas, other soft drinks, such as Mountain Dew, and some bottled water, such as Cup of Joe.

- Don't take No-Doz. Avoid alcoholic beverages at dinnertime and during the rest of the evening, too. Even though alcohol is a sedative, it can disrupt sleep.

- Don't take over-the-counter sleeping pills or friends' or relatives' sleeping pills. Only take sleep medicine with your health care provider's permission.

- Count sheep! Picturing a repeated image may bore you to sleep.

Lifestyle Issues

Tobacco Use

"When I was a student at the University of Michigan, I was a 2 pack a day Marlboro smoker. Luckily, my psychology professor suggested I design a stop smoking program to help me fulfill a class assignment as well as to help me become smoke-free. Not only did I successfully quit, but it launched me into a career in health promotion. It was the best thing I have ever done."

Don R. Powell, Ph.D.,
Founder and President of the American Institute for Preventive Medicine and author of this guide.

Benefits of Quitting

Smoking is our nation's #1 preventable cause of illness and premature death. Over 400,000 people in the U.S. die each year from the effects of smoking.

You may not worry about getting lung cancer, emphysema, and/or heart disease, because if one or more of these occur, it will be 30 to 40 years down the road. These illnesses may not motivate you to quit, but they should! Smoking is one of the worst things you can do for your health! If health benefits don't make you want to quit smoking, focus on the immediate benefits of quitting. These include:

- Fresher breath. Each year, smoking a pack-a-day puts 1 cup of tar into your lungs. The tobacco tar causes bad breath.

- Cleaner smelling hair and clothes.

- Saving money. (See "**The Cost of $moking**" on page 89.)

- Fresher looking skin. Nicotine narrows blood vessels which decreases blood flow. In the face, the result is premature wrinkling. After as little as 5 years of smoking, your face could show these wrinkles, known as "smoker's face."

- Improved stamina. After smoking a few packs of cigarettes or several cigars, your blood can contain up to 15 times more carbon monoxide (the same poisonous gas in car exhaust) than a nonsmoker's blood. Carbon monoxide robs the body of oxygen causing a slower reaction time and impaired energy, strength, and coordination.

- Improved sexual performance. Males who smoke have a more difficult time maintaining erections and have a lower sperm count. Female smokers have a higher rate of infertility.

Smokers' Excuses

Six common reasons smokers use to explain why they smoke and why their reasons are incorrect are listed below and on page 89.

- *I'll gain weight if I quit.* After quitting, the average smoker gains between 4 to 10 pounds. Nicotine raises metabolism, which increases the amount of calories used. After quitting, metabolism slows down to a normal level. Exercise and healthy eating can stop most, if not all, of this weight gain.

- *I need cigarettes to relax.* Nicotine is actually a stimulant; it prompts the nervous system and the adrenal glands to trigger the release of adrenaline, the "fight or flight" hormone. Adrenaline leaves you feeling wired, not relaxed.

- *I know lots of people who smoke. They're still healthy.* We all know people like this, but they're the exception rather than the rule. The odds are stacked against you.

Tobacco Use, *Continued*

- *Cigarettes won't hurt me. I'm in good shape.* Don't bet on it. Even if you don't die from smoking, you'll almost certainly have health problems, such as trouble breathing, a hacking cough, high blood pressure, or heart disease. Quit now, before the damage is done!

- *I've tried to quit dozens of times. It's no use.* If you've tried to quit smoking 8 times, and failed 8 times, each try increases the chance that you'll succeed. Most ex-smokers tried many times before they quit for good.

- *I can't imagine life without cigarettes.* You weren't born smoking; you picked up the habit. You lived before you smoked. You'll live after you quit. And you'll probably live longer!

Bidis – Not a Safe Alternative

Bidis are small brown flavored cigarettes made in India. They are cheaper and easier to buy than regular cigarettes. They are also dangerous.

One bidi produces more than 3 times the carbon monoxide and nicotine than one cigarette and more than 5 times the amount of tar than one cigarette.

In India, bidi-making employs about 5 million women and an estimated 325,000 children a year, at wages as low as $.80 per day. Many rollers suffer from lung disease from inhaling the tobacco dust.

The High Cost of Cigarettes

The boxes below show the minimum amount you can save if you quit smoking now. The figures are based on a cost of $6.00 per pack. The totals don't include the interest you would earn if you put this money in the bank. To see how much cigarettes cost you, access www.cancer.org and search for "Calculate the Cost of Smoking,"

The Cost of $moking			
	Number of Packs a Day		
	1	2	3
Day	$6.00	$12.00	$18.00
Week	$42.00	$84.00	$126.00
Month	$180.00	$360.00	$540.00
Year	$2,190.00	$4,380.00	$6,570.00
10 Years	$21,900.00	$43,800.00	$65,700.00
20 Years	$43,800.00	$87,600.00	$131,400.00
30 Years	$65,700.00	$131,400.00	$197,100.00
40 Years	$87,600.00	$175,200.00	$262,800.00

Lifestyle Issues

Tobacco Use, *Continued*

Snuff Out Smokeless Tobacco

Regardless of whether you smoke it, chew it, or just place it between your cheek and gums, all forms of tobacco are hazardous to your health. "Snuff" and chewing tobacco were once considered safe alternatives to cigarettes. They're not. If you use smokeless tobacco, you absorb nicotine through the mucous membrane of your mouth. Nicotine absorbed in this way is no less addictive than nicotine inhaled from cigarettes or cigars. If you use smokeless tobacco, you run a high risk of: Cancers of the mouth, esophagus, larynx, and stomach; a precancerous condition called leukoplakia (a whitish, wrinkling of the mouth lining); heart disease; gum disease; and tooth decay.

The best way to avoid these risks, of course, is to never use smokeless tobacco. But if you already use it, here are some suggestions to help you stop:

- Ignore the appeals of sports figures who promote smokeless tobacco in advertisements.

- Use substitutes, such as gum, mints, or toothpicks, etc.

- Distract yourself with other activities.

- Reward yourself each day you don't chew tobacco.

Medications That Can Help

Some tobacco users who are addicted to nicotine find it easier to quit smoking using nicotine reduction therapy. This includes using a nicotine patch (e.g., Nicoderm, Nicotrol), a nicotine gum (e.g., Nicorette), or nicotine lozenges (e.g., Commit). These little doses of nicotine let them reduce their nicotine cravings and wean themselves from tobacco with less anxiety and irritability. The patch, gum, and lozenges are available over-the-counter. A nicotine nasal spray (e.g., Nicotrol NS) and a nicotine inhaler (e.g., Nicotrol) are available by prescription.

Other prescribed medications, such as Chantix and Zyban, do not contain nicotine, but alters brain chemistry to help reduce tobacco cravings.

Also, studies have shown that combining a stop smoking medication with behavior modification greatly increases your chances for success. Get help and step-by-step guides to quit from the Web site listed below.

For Information, Contact:

American Lung Association
800.LUNG.USA (586-4872)
www.lungusa.org

National Network of Tobacco Cessation Quitlines
800.QUIT.NOW (784.8669)

Smokefree.gov
www.smokefree.gov

Lifestyle Issues

Sexual Health

Closeness, touching, and intimacy are good for health. One way to experience these is through sexual contact. Some people decide to delay sex until they are in a long-term, committed relationship. Others decide to become sexually active without one. If you choose to be sexually active, consider your health and peace of mind by using "safer sex."

Safer Sex to Help Prevent STIs

Safer sex means being intimate, but using measures that minimize the risk of sexually transmitted infections (STIs). Not having sex, including intercourse, oral sex, anal sex, and genital-to-genital contact is the only sure way to eliminate the risk for STIs. Caressing, hugging, dry kissing, and masturbation are no risk or extremely low-risk practices. So is limiting your sexual contact to one person your entire life if your partner is also monogamous and does not have an STI.

■ Latex and polyurethane condoms can help reduce the risk of spreading HIV infection and may reduce the risk for other STIs. To do this, they must be used the right way for every sex act. Sex with condoms isn't totally "safe sex," but is "less risky" sex. Use condoms with "prevent disease" on the package label. Barriers made of natural membranes, such as lamb skin, do not offer effective protection against STIs. Unless you are in a monogamous relationship in which neither you nor your partner has an STI, carry latex condoms and insist that they be used every time you have genital-to-genital contact and/or oral sex. If you or your partner is allergic to latex, use polyurethane condoms.

■ For oral-vaginal sex and oral-anal sex, use latex dams ("doilies"). These are latex squares.

■ Using latex condoms with spermicides, such as nonoxynol-9 (N-9), are no more effective than other lubricated condoms in protecting against HIV and other STIs. Using spermicides with N-9 are not effective in preventing chlamydia, cervical gonorrhea, or HIV infection. Don't use spermicides alone to prevent STIs/HIV. Also, using spermicides with N-9 often has been linked with genital lesions which may be associated with an increased risk of HIV transmission. In addition, N-9 may increase the risk for HIV transmission during anal intercourse. If you need to use lubricants, use water-based ones, such as K-Y Brand Jelly. *Don't use oil-based or "petroleum" ones, such as Vaseline. They can damage latex barriers.*

■ Don't have sex while under the influence of drugs or alcohol.

■ Limit sexual partners. Sexual contact with many persons increases the risk for STIs, especially if no protection is used.

■ Discuss a new partner's sexual history with him or her before you begin a sexual relationship. (Be aware, though, that persons are not always honest about their sexual history.)

■ Avoid sexual contact with persons whose health status and health practices are not known.

Lifestyle Issues

Sexual Health, *Continued*

- Avoid sex if either partner has signs and symptoms of a genital infection, such as sores or a discharge.

- Wash the genitals with soap and water before and after sexual intercourse.

- After manual sexual contact in another person's genital area, wash your hands with hot water and an antibacterial soap, especially before you touch your eyes or anyone else's genitals.

- Talk to your health care provider about getting vaccinated for hepatitis B.

- Follow your health care provider's advice to check for STIs.

If you have multiple sex partners, you may be advised to check for STIs every 6 months, even if you don't have any symptoms.

Seek treatment for a sexually transmitted infection if you suspect or know your sex partner is infected. Your sexual partner(s) should also be contacted and treated.

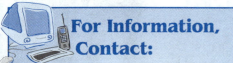

For Information, Contact:

Your schools' Student Health Center, your health care provider, or your local health department

CDC National STD Hotline
800.CDC.INFO (232.4636)

American Sexual Health Association (ASHA)
919.361.8488
www.ashastd.org

Sexual Assault

Sexual assault is an unlawful act that may involve the touching of intimate body parts, sexual intimidation, or forced sexual penetration. This includes sexual intercourse, oral sex, and digital penetration. Rape is forced sexual intercourse. Force may be by verbal threats, physical restraint, or violence. Stalking is defined as repeated, obsessive, fear-inducing behavior that makes the victim afraid or concerned for his or her safety.

A study funded by the Department of Justice found that sexual assault and stalking of college females are widespread and grossly underestimated. U.S. statistics report:

- About 3% of coeds are raped during each academic year. Over the course of 5 calendar years, including summers and vacations, 20-25% may be raped.

- Nationally, an additional 15.5% of college females are sexually victimized (e.g., sexual contact is completed with force or threat of non-physical force, threat of rape, or threat of contact).

- Nationally, 13.1% of coeds are stalked an average of 60 days during an academic year.

- Nationally, less than 5% of completed and attempted rapes of college females are reported to the police or campus officials. About 67% of the victims tell a friend.

Sexual Health, *Continued*

- Nine out of 10 victims knew their assailant. {*Note:* Almost all sexual assaults on college campuses are acquaintance rapes and, in most cases, at least one of the persons involved is under the influence of alcohol or another drug.}

- Between 3 and 6% of male university students reported being raped and up to 25% reported being sexually assaulted. Only about 1% of male rape victims reported it to the police.

Safety Tips to Reduce the Chances for Sexual Assault

Be aware of the risks of date rape with drinking alcohol. About 75% of male students who take part in acquaintance rape had been drinking; about 55% of female students had.

- The best defense is to not drink. If you drink, limit alcohol intake.

- Don't drink anything you have not brought or opened yourself. Don't drink from another person's container, from a punch bowl, beer bong, etc. When at a bar or club, accept drinks only from a bartender or waiter.

- Keep your drink in your hand and under your watch at all times. If needed, have a friend watch your drink. Do the same for your friend(s).

- Don't drink alcohol in a high-risk setting for sexual assault (e.g., frat house or team parties or with persons you don't know and/or trust).

Be aware of these "date-rape" drugs, which have no odor or color when mixed with drinks:

- Rohypnol. See the Drug Chart under "**Drugs & Drug Safety**" on page 72 for the effects of this drug which can last 6 to 8 hours. This drug is added to drinks and punches at parties, raves, etc., usually to lower sexual inhibitions in females. When mixed with alcohol or other drugs, Rohypnol can cause death.

- GHB and GLB. See the Drug Chart under "**Drugs & Drug Safety**" on page 71 for the effects of this drug which last about 8 hours. If you have had this drug, you may wake up partially clothed with no recollection of a sexual assault. GHB is often made in homes with recipes and ingredients found and purchased on the Internet. GHB can cause death.

Consider using a coaster or test strip made to detect date rape drugs in drinks before you take a sip. An example is Drink Safe Coaster™ by Drink Safe Technology. For information, contact www.drinksafetech.com.

If you suspect you have been drugged, keep a sample of your drink. Get help immediately. Have a friend help you get medical care. Call EMS, if necessary. Get tested for the drug within 12 hours of the suspected incident at a hospital emergency department.

Do not have sex with a person who is under the influence of alcohol and/or drugs which compromise consent. Also, look out for the safety of your friends and yourself and don't put yourself in vulnerable situations.

Lifestyle Issues

Sexual Health, *Continued*

- Alert your female friends (and the authorities) to rumors of guys using date-rape drugs.

- Don't assume that anyone under the influence is "too nice a guy" to commit sexual assault. Intervene on a friend's behalf (e.g., walk her out of a party, take her to a safe place, etc.).

- Know your sexual limitations and communicate them both verbally and nonverbally. If you sense you are being pressured to have sex and don't want to, state your position clearly. Say "NO" emphatically when you mean "NO!" Be aware, too, that a female/partner does not need to say the word "NO" to mean "NO." Listen for words like, "I'm just not ready," "We're going too fast," etc. The female/partner may be afraid to say "NO."

- Attend your school's classes, etc. on preventing acquaintance rape, sexual assault, etc. Take a class in self-defense.

- Carry a cell phone with you to call for help, if needed.

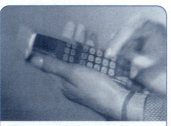

Carry a cell phone with you to call for help, if needed.

- Avoid being alone, especially in unsafe situations and with strangers and persons you don't know well or feel safe with.

- Keep the doors to your home and car locked. Don't open doors to strangers. Don't tell strangers that you are alone.

If Rape Occurs

- Do not shower, clean or wash up in any way, or change clothing before you go to the hospital emergency department. Doing so could destroy evidence (e.g., blood type, hair samples, etc.) which may not be legally acceptable if collected later than 72 hours after the rape. If you have removed clothes worn at the time of the rape, put them in a paper bag and take them with you to the E.R.

- Get medical or police help right away. (Date-rape drugs may not be detectable after 12 hours.) Go to the E.R. Recall and write down as many details as you can. Report the rapist's age, height, weight, race, hair color, clothing worn, noticeable body marks, tattoos, etc. If a vehicle was involved, report its type, color, license plate, etc. Take a friend with you for comfort and support. At the E.R., you will get information about health care providers in your area who can help you after the E.R. visit. You will likely need their services at some point.

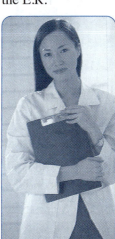

If a rape occurs, go to a hospital ER.

- Talk to the emergency care provider about emergency contraception and tests for STIs.

- Contact your campus Sexual Assault Crisis Center or call the Rape Crisis Hotline at 800.656.HOPE (4673).

Lifestyle Issues

Sexual Health, *Continued*

Birth Control Options

Discuss these and additional methods that meet your needs with your health care provider. More than one method may be needed to prevent pregnancy <u>and</u> HIV/STIs. If no method is used, the chance of pregnancy is 85 to 90%. Percent failure rate is the number of pregnancies expected per 100 females per year.

- **Abstinence.** No sexual intercourse between a female and a male. 0% failure rate for pregnancy and HIV/STIs.

- **Birth Control Patch.** Hormones from a prescribed patch worn on the skin weekly for 3 weeks; not worn the 4th week. 1% failure rate. Does not prevent HIV/STIs.

- **Birth Control Pills.** Prescribed hormones in pill form. 3% failure rate. Many options. Do not prevent HIV/STIs. Some medicines can make the pill less effective.

- **Cervical Cap.** Prescribed plastic cap placed over the opening of the cervix. Used with spermicide. 16% failure rate for females who have not given birth; 32% for females who have. Does not prevent HIV/STIs.

- **Condom (Female).** Over-the-counter (OTC) polyurethane barrier placed inside the vagina. 21% failure rate. May give some protection against HIV/STIs. Should not be used at same time with a male condom.

- **Condom (Male).** OTC latex or polyurethane sheath worn over an erect penis. 11% failure rate. Latex condoms help protect against gonorrhea, syphilis, and HIV and are more durable than ones made of animal membranes, which do not prevent HIV/STIs.

- **Depo-Provera.** Prescribed hormones given through a shot every 3 months. Less than 1% failure rate. Does not prevent HIV/STIs.

- **Diaphragm.** Prescribed reusable, thin, soft, rubber cap that covers the cervix. Used with spermicide. 17% failure rate. Does not protect against HIV. May help protect against chlamydia, gonorrhea, and trichomoniasis.

- **Emergency Hormonal Contraception Pills or IUD Insertion.** Prescribed pills need to be started within 72 hours; IUD within 7 days after unprotected sex. About 11-25% failure rate for pills (the sooner taken, the more effective); less than 1% for IUD. Neither prevent HIV/STIs.

- **FemCap®.** Prescribed silicone rubber device that fits snugly over the cervix. 14% failure rate for females who have not given birth; 29% for females who have. Does not prevent HIV/STIs.

- **Implanon®.** Thin plastic implant that releases the hormone progestin for up to 3 years. Less than 1% failure rate. Does not prevent HIV/STIs.

- **Intrauterine Device (IUD).** Small copper device inserted into uterus (and needs to be removed) by a health care provider. Can remain in place up to 12 years. Less than 1% failure rate. Does not prevent HIV/STIs.

- **Intrauterine System (IUS).** Mirena®, a device placed in uterus by health care provider. Can remain in place for 5 years. 8% failure rate. Does not prevent HIV/STIs.

- **Lea's Shield®.** Prescribed silicone rubber device that fits snugly over the cervix. Used with spermicide. 15% failure rate. Does not prevent HIV/STIs.

Lifestyle Issues

Sexual Health, *Continued*

- **Natural Family Planning (Fertility Awareness, Periodic Abstinence).** Sex must be limited to "safe days." About 20% failure rate. Does not prevent HIV/STIs.

- **NuvaRing®.** Prescribed soft, flexible ring that a female inserts deep into the vagina. The ring stays in place for 3 weeks; is removed the week of menstrual period. 1% failure rate. Does not prevent HIV/STIs.

- **Spermicides (Foams, Jellies, Creams, etc.).** OTC chemicals inserted into the vagina that kill sperm before it enters the uterus. 15-21% failure rate. More reliable when used with barrier methods (condoms, diaphragms). Inserted between 5 and 90 minutes before intercourse. Need to reapply for repeated acts of intercourse.

- **Sterilization (Female).** Surgical or nonsurgical, permanent form of birth control to burn, cut, tie off, or block the fallopian tubes. Less than 1% failure rate. Does not prevent HIV/STIs.

- **Sterilization (Male).** Vasectomy. The tubes (vas deferens) through which sperm travels from the testes are cut. Less than 1% failure rate. Does not prevent HIV/STIs.

- **Today® Sponge.** OTC polyurethane foam barrier that contains spermicide. Must be left in place for 6 hours after last intercourse, but should not be worn more than 24 hours after sex. 9-19% failure rate. Gives some protection for STIs.

- **Withdrawal.** Removal of the penis before ejaculation. Up to 27% failure rate. Does not prevent HIV/STIs. Control of ejaculation is necessary and sperm may leak before this occurs.

Signs of Pregnancy

- Missed menstrual periods. {*Note:* Stress or illness can cause a period to be late, too. And, some females do not have regular periods. It may be hard for them to know if their period is 2 weeks late. Other females can have a light menstrual period or spotting and still be pregnant. So watch for other signs also listed here.}

- Abnormal vaginal bleeding.

- Breast tenderness, swelling, and/or tingling.

- The dark areas around the nipples are darker than before and the tiny glands around the nipples stick up.

- Feeling tired.

- Nausea or vomiting.

- Frequent urination.

- Unusual food cravings or your taste for certain foods changes; a metallic taste in the mouth.

- Mood swings.

- Slight elevation in body temperature.

- Acne due to extra-active oil glands.

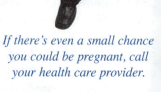

If there's even a small chance you could be pregnant, call your health care provider.